Preface

What does detox mean to me?
Detoxification to me means being free from all threats: physical, psychological, and environmental alike. It means being healed from not only the toxins I digest within my diet, but being relieved from all of the toxic relationships, and having the ability to feel like I can remove all types of waste from my life.

Why do we need to detox?
After just 24 hours toxins can already exceed the body's threshold depending on where you've gone, what you've eaten, and and what you've touched!

Therefore it is important to be cautious and start to eliminate toxins as soon as we have the opportunity! This process will help reduce risk of illness and morbidity.

What is detoxing?
People normally associate detoxing as a process that cleanses organs. However, detoxing facilitates cleansing of accumulated waste from our cells. This occurs within the organs, and the result is better organ function because when cells are clear and free of debris and excess organic compounds, they can function better.

Disclaimer from Liability

The information provided by Discover Your Greatest Self ("we," "us" or "our") on http://www.jasmineblake.com (the "Site"), through guides, books, content, courses, or programs, and our mobile application is for general informational purposes only. All information on the site, guides, books, content, courses, or programs, and our mobile application is provided in good faith, and use references to cite all claims. However, we make no representation or warranty of any kind, express or implied, regarding the accuracy, adequacy, validity, reliability, availability or completeness of any information on the site, guides, books, content, courses, or programs, or our mobile application. Under NO circumstance shall we have any liability to you for any loss or damage of any kind incurred as a result of the use of the site, guides, books, content, courses, or programs, or our mobile application or reliance on any information provided on the site and our mobile application. Your use of the site, guides, books, content, courses, or programs, and our mobile application and your reliance on any information on the site, guides, books, content, courses, or programs, and our mobile application is solely at your own risk.

Warning:
"Health information in this booklet is provided for general information to the public and for educational purposes only and is not a substitute for professional physicians' medical advice or medical diagnosing. You're liable for all risks for the use, misuse, non-use, or reliance of this information."

Second Edition

ISBN:9781943117369 (Electronic Edition)
ISBN:9781943117130 (Print Edition)
ISBN:9781943117260 (Print Edition)

Copyright © 2019 by:
Discover Your Greatest Self™ a True Paleo, Inc. company
All rights reserved.

No part of this book may be reproduced in any form; or by any electronic, mechanical or any other means including information storage and retrieval systems without expressed permission in writing from the publisher or Jasmine Blake, except by reviewers who may quote passages in their review.

Editing by:
EatitUP™ Editing Team

Primary Author:
Dr. Jasmine Blake Hollywood, DCN, LDN, CNS, BA-Psy, CRPS, ORDM

Co-Author:
Dr. Miriam Whitfield, DCN, CPT

Printed, written, and bound in United States

Published by:
Discover Your Greatest Self™

True Paleo Inc™
PO Box 130282
Tampa, Fl. 33681
www.jasmineblake.com

Table of Contents

Introduction	1
Free Radicals	5
Water	10
Detoxification Organs	14
Phases of Detoxification	19
Antioxidants	24
Nutrients	28
Nutritional Methods	35
How do we detox?	43
Detoxes and Remedies	48
Meal Plans and Menus	52
Recipes	59
Extras	70
References	73

Introduction

Understanding Detoxification

One challenge confronted by society lies in the inclination to embrace information given to us by media sources. Our perception of detoxification has been molded into a specific framework, fostering stereotypes that lead to confusion in comprehending it's true essence. Consequently, the objective of this book is to elucidate the meaning of "detox" and provide an understanding of the workings of the body's detoxification process.

Defining Detoxification

In history, both doctors of medicine and philosophy have tried to define detoxing. The standard definition of detoxification is *the process or period of time in which an individual abstains from or rids the body of toxic or unhealthy substances.*

The Metabolic Pathway of Detoxing

According to researchers, detoxification is characterized as a *metabolic pathway*. This pathway is committed to eliminating xenobiotics, free radicals, and other accumulated toxins from our cells. As toxins build up, our well-being is compromised, prompting a natural inclination to eliminate them for improved health. This organic detoxification process mirrors our human nature. As our bodies attempt to remove waste from our cells, our organs are afforded an opportunity to operate more efficiently. Facilitating this process can be achieved through practices like increased water intake, targeted nutrient consumption, and stress reduction.

Where do toxins come from?

The sources of toxins are diverse and encompass several avenues. Toxins can originate from the foods we consume, the beverages we drink, environmental pollutants the chemicals present in our daily-use products, personal hygiene products, kitchenware, and even stress. In essence, toxins are substances that are alien to the body, lacking recognition or utility within the body's functions.

Substance Use and Drug Addiction

Over the decades, the concept of detoxing has been misunderstood as a means of recovering from narcotics. For many, this practice is closely linked to the withdrawal process associated with addictive substances. It's important to note that all types of drugs, including certain plant compounds, fall under this category. As these substances accumulate within our cells, they can trigger a toxic overload phenomenon. This, in turn, can disrupt cellular communication, leading to mood imbalances and various other complications. Over time, our bodies may become accustomed to this altered state, potentially leading to dependency on these substances.

Introduction

Weight Loss
In recent decades, detoxification has gained significant popularity due to media promotion of it as a weight loss method. This trend led to the widespread adoption of plant-based blends, health beverages, and various over-the-counter products aimed at facilitating weight loss through detox. Unfortunately, this approach to detoxification has often been misused and can result in adverse health effects. Presently, the perception of detox remains linked to extreme weight loss practices in the public consciousness.

Detoxification Phases
The detoxification process comprises distinct phases, each involving specific organs and nutrients to facilitate the elimination of toxins. Occasionally, one phase may prove more effective than another, resulting in an imbalance that hinders the body's ability to expel particular substances. Furthermore, this malfunction can create challenges in effectively clearing certain compounds. Additionally, genetic predispositions play a role in influencing the various phases of detoxification, further impacting the efficiency of this intricate process.

Why should people detox regularly?
Regular detoxification is important because toxins place significant strain on our cells. As cells work harder to counteract the effects of toxins, they experience accelerated aging and eventual breakdown. This cellular decline subsequently impacts the functioning of our organs. When our organs begin to malfunction, our bodies manifest signs of disease. Over time, untreated diseases can accumulate and contribute to serious health issues, potentially leading to mortality. Detoxifying regularly can help alleviate this burden on our cells and organs, promoting overall well-being and longevity.

How do we know when we need to detox?
Recognizing the need for detoxification relies on observing certain health outcomes and symptoms that arise from the continuous accumulation of toxins within our bodies. These symptoms might manifest as constipation, fatigue, headaches, unexplained weight gain, or a general sense of discomfort. Often, we may not be aware of toxin build up until our organs exhibit serious distress signals. Researchers are increasingly connecting current states of disease to the accumulation of toxins. Conditions such as cancer, hormone imbalances, type 2 diabetes, and neurological disorders have been associated with toxin overload. This underscores the significance of maintaining a nutritious, stress-free lifestyle to mitigate the risks posed by toxin accumulation.

What is "Lifestyle Toxicity"?
Lifestyle toxicity encompasses various forms of toxicity that affect our bodies on a physiological level. Detoxification is often associated with the removal of

tangible substances like mold, drugs, alcohol, sugars, dietary components, and air pollutants. However, toxins extend beyond the physical realm. Toxicity can permeate various aspects of life, including thoughts, jobs, and relationships. While these forms of toxicity may be overlooked, their impact can be profound, and many individuals suffer the consequences of failing to eliminate these toxins from their lives. This concept is closely related to mental and spiritual health imbalances that are more commonly recognized. Toxic lifestyles can lead to disturbances in mental and emotional well-being, distorted perceptions, an imbalanced biofield, and feelings of isolation.

A Common Practice
Detoxing can be done as a daily practice by just simply incorporating it into your lifestyle. It can be done sporadically throughout the year by adding your regimen to meal plans, as a part of your religion, or by using it regularly throughout the fasting technique. There are many different remedies and recipes for successful detoxing. So, let's dive in!

Free Radicals

From a scientific perspective, much of what exists in the natural world eventually will pair to something else through the phenomenon of magnetism. This natural attraction is governed by magnetic fields, which play a pivotal role in existence, including sources of light. or simple physical and chemical reactions. The concept of magnetic polarity is described as the *orientation of two poles*, commonly referred to as the 'north' and 'south' poles. with opposing poles exhibiting an attractive force that leads to their eventual pairing, creating a rotational effect.

A similar principle applies to the molecular composition present in all life forms. Atoms within the human body possess a natural magnetic polarity, characterized by positive or negative charges. It's this inherent polarity that draws atoms together. When molecules or atoms come close enough to each other, they form bonds, potentially altering their charge or enhancing it. This process of attraction governs molecular rotation and triggers crucial biochemical reactions, which are essential for sustaining human life (Phaniendra et al., 2015; Zhang et al., 2015).

In the absence of a magnetic field, the alignment of polar molecules becomes random, rendering the pairing of positive and negative charges impossible. Similarly, non-polar molecules without a magnetic field exhibit random movements. Molecules that move at random or have random 'spins' (ie. rotations), are referred to as *free radicals* (Phaniendra et al., 2015). In definition, *free radicals are atoms, molecules, or ions that have unpaired valence electrons* (Zhang et al., 2015). Interactions between external magnetic forces and electron spins, governs these reactions, highlighting the intricate relationship between magnetism and biochemical processes (Zhang et al., 2015).

Radical pairs often emerge as short-lived intermediates, generated through processes such as decomposition, electron transfer, or hydrogen transfer reactions from singlet or triplet excited atomic states (Zhang et al., 2015). However, the presence of these molecules within the human body carries potential risks. These highly reactive molecules can seize electrons from other molecules to maintain their magnetic or polar equilibrium, triggering a chain reaction (Phaniendra et al., 2015). This process causes previously stable molecules to transform into free radicals, setting off a sequence that can lead to cellular damaged (Phaniendra et al., 2015). Over time, as this damage accumulates, cells become compromised, ultimately culminating in cell death. This cascading effect of free radicals impacts various biomolecules such as biolipids, proteins, carbohydrates, and DNA, contributing to the onset of contemporary diseases (Al-Mamary & Moussa, 2021; Lobo et al., 2010; Phaniendra et al., 2015).

Reactive Oxygen Species

Reactive Oxygen Species (ROS), encompassing both free radical and non-free radical derivatives of oxygen, are integral components within the human body due to the constant inhalation of oxygen, essential for sustaining life (Phaniendra et al., 2015). Yet, the presence of oxygen derivatives can also pose substantial threats to human health, underscoring the necessity of mitigating free radical oxygen derivatives for longevity (Phaniendra et al., 2015).

Oxygen exhibits what could be called "paralleled spin". Its unpaired electrons rotate in the same direction. This characteristic impedes oxygen's interaction with its opposite, as the opposite electron would have to spin in the opposite direction to pair. Additionally, oxygen cannot accept two electrons simultaneously, leading to the formation of a substance called superoxide (Al-Mamary & Moussa, 2021). This transformation transpires within the mitochondria (Al-Mamary & Moussa, 2021).

Superoxide is recognized as a detrimental form of oxygen, marked by its heightened reactivity and damaging potential, often termed as a free radical of ROS (Al-Mamary & Moussa, 2021). Other compounds also have the potential to transform into ROS, including hydroxyl, peroxyl radicals, singlet oxygen, ozone, and hypochlorous acid, stemming from various biochemical reactions (Al-Mamary & Moussa, 2021; Phaniendra et al., 2015). Notably, the superoxide molecule can further convert into hydrogen peroxide, triggering the formation of other free radicals such as *hydroxyl* and *peroxyl* radicals (Al-Mamary & Moussa, 2021; Phaniendra et al., 2015). Singlet oxygen is generated through cataclysmic reactions involving lipoxygenases, dioxygenases, and lactoperoxidase, while ozone results from water oxidation, and hypochlorous acid emerges from hydrogen peroxide reactions and chlorination (Al-Mamary & Moussa, 2021; Phaniendra et al., 2015).

Diverse types of ROS include:

Superoxide	$O_2^{\cdot-}$
Hydroxyl	$OH^{\cdot}$
Alkoxyl	$RO^{\cdot}$
Peroxyl	$ROO^{\cdot}$
Hydrogen Peroxide	H_2O_2
Singlet Oxygen	$^1O_2$
Ozone	O_3
Organic peroxide	ROOH
Hypochlorous acid	HOCl
Hypobromous acid	HOBr

Reactive Nitrogen Species

Reactive Nitrogen Species (RNS), encompassing both free radical and non-free radical derivatives of nitrogen and oxygen, share mechanistic similarities with ROS (Al-Mamary & Moussa, 2021; Phaniendra et al., 2015).

The diverse types of RNS include:

Nitric oxide	NOO·
Nitrogen dioxide	NO$_2$·
Peroxynitrite	ONOO–
Nitrosyl cation	NO+
Nitroxyl anion	NO–
Dinitrogen trioxide	N2O3
Dinitrogen tetraoxide	N2O4
Nitrous acid	HNO2
Peroxynitrous acid	ONOOH
Nitryl chloride	NO2Cl

Just like ROS, RNS can have detrimental effects on cellular components. These species have been associated with numerous pathological conditions, including inflammation, neurodegenerative disorders, cardiovascular diseases, and cancer (Al-Mamary & Moussa, 2021; Phaniendra et al., 2015).

Free radicals, both ROS and RNS, are indeed considered toxins! Their presence in the body can lead to cellular damage, particularly impacting lipids, proteins, carbohydrates, and DNA within mitochondria (Al-Mamary & Moussa, 2021; Lobo et al., 2010; Phaniendra et al., 2015). The damaging effects of ROS are particularly pronounced on DNA due to its proximity to ROS production sites (Phaniendra et al., 2015). RNA is comparatively weaker than DNA and more susceptible to damage (Phaniendra et al., 2015). Moreover, lipid membranes are vulnerable to damage from carbon-centered lipid and lipid peroxyl radicals, while proteins within the cell can become denatured in the presence of free radicals (Phaniendra et al., 2015).

Sources of Free Radicals

Internal Sources	External Sources
Phagocytosis	Ozone
Inflammation from immune system	Chemicals
Oxygen	Cigarette smoke
Peroxisomes	Radiation
Arachidonate pathways	Environmental pollutants
Xanthine oxidase	Exercise
	Drugs

Oxidative Stress

Oxidative Stress, often referred to as the result of excessive free radical activity, emerges when an imbalance occurs between free radicals and

Free radicals

antioxidants within the body (Lobo et al., 2010). This imbalance leads to an accumulation of radical molecules that the body struggles to eliminate promptly, resulting in an overload of toxins. The inability to efficiently clear these toxins contributes to oxidative stress, which, if left unchecked, can accelerate the aging process (Lobo et al., 2010).

Aging cells are notably affected by the impact of free radicals, which are believed to increase in prevalence as individuals age (Lobo et al., 2010). Additionally, free radicals are implicated in the onset of various diseases, the nature of which is influenced by a combination of genetic predisposition and environmental factors (Lobo et al., 2010). Furthermore, ROS's influence on the promotion of carcinogenesis and its significant role in shaping cardiovascular disease outcomes have been extensively documented (Lobo et al., 2010).

Water

Free radicals

Detoxifying Properties of Water
The dance of molecules involves a continuous spin, and for free radicals, their orbital completion hinges on extracting hydrogen, oxygen, or halogen atoms from other molecules within the body—an act akin to molecular theft. Yet, free radicals aren't one-sided thieves; they must also relinquish hydrogen or oxygen atoms at times. Herein lies the importance of water consumption.

In the modern world, we're surrounded by various fluids, but the fundamental truth remains: without water, survival beyond 3-4 days is a precarious proposition. Water, with its intrinsic attributes, holds a vital place in our existence.

Potential of Hydrogen (pH)
One of water's defining characteristics is its pH measurement, which gauges its acidity or alkalinity. This metric is grounded in the concentration of free hydrogen and hydroxyl ions within water. Higher hydronium ions denote greater acidity, while an abundance of hydroxyl ions indicates alkalinity.

The pH scale spans from 0 to 14, with 7 marking neutrality. A pH below 7 signals acidity, while a pH exceeding 7 signifies an alkaline environment. The spectrum encapsulates the vast range of pH levels that substances, including water, can exhibit.

Figure 1: *pH Scale*

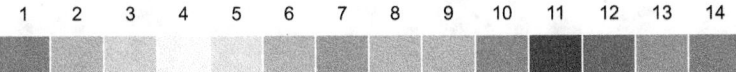

0. Battery acid
1. Stomach acid
2. Vinegar, lemon juice
3. Grapefruit juice, soda
4. Tomato, oranges, kimchi
5. Black coffee
6. Urine, milk, saliva, rain water
7. Water, blood
8. Seawater
9. Baking soda
10. Indigestion tablet, detergent
11. Ammonia
12. Soapy water
13. Bleach, oven cleaner, lye
14. Drain cleaner

Free radicals

It is reported that the more alkaline the water is humans drink the more it detoxifies free radicals. The theory behind this is that as the alkalinity of water increases, so does its capacity to scavenge free radicals, neutralizing toxins. In essence, this process acts as a protective shield against these potentially harmful molecules.

Importance of pH

The more acidic a substance is, the more damage it does. Acids corrode and damage things they come into contact with. Nonetheless, strong bases (ie. high alkalinity) and substances are also caustic and can severely damage things it comes into contact with.

This prompts a pivotal question: does alkaline water actually help or harm us?

Hydroxyls, mentioned in the previous chapter, are free radicals, generated when a water molecule loses a hydrogen atom. Hydroxyls make things more alkaline However, a substance's level of alkalinity is determined by the ratio of negatively charged hydroxyls to positively charged hydroniums. If negatively charged hydroxyls outnumber positively charged hydroniums, the substance becomes more basic. Conversely, if positively charged hydroniums exceed negatively charged hydroxyls, the substance leans towards acidity. The balance between hydroxyl and hydronium ions establishes neutrality.

Figure 2: *Hydroxyl Reaction*

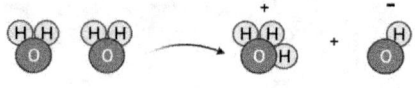

water (H_2O)   hydronium (H_3O)   hydroxyl (HO)   the body?

Hydroxyl molecules rank among the most destructive radicals within the human body (Al-Mamary & Moussa, 2021). However, their single hydrogen atom leaves the door open for further atom bonding. Compounds with multiple hydroxyl groups are termed polyhydroxylated (Al-Mamary & Moussa, 2021). These compounds have the capacity to donate an electron or a hydrogen free radical to molecules that would otherwise trigger free radical formation due to their inability to scavenge electrons or hydrogen radicals (Al-Mamary & Moussa, 2021). This donation process effectively thwarts free radical generation (Al-Mamary & Moussa, 2021).

Phenolic compounds like flavonoids are examples of molecules containing multiple hydroxyl groups (Al-Mamary & Moussa, 2021). Hydrogen-rich water,

Water

characterized by its alkaline pH and abundance of negative hydroxyl molecules, can donate electrons and hydrogen radicals to other free radicals seeking pairing opportunities.

Intriguingly, geographical variations impact pH levels, with the northwestern part of the US more alkaline, the southeastern part less alkaline, and the northeastern part most acidic. Therefore, living in the north west is healthier for humans. This intriguing facet underlines the potential health benefits of residing in alkaline-rich environments.

Note: The fun fact and information source provided have been adopted from the National Atmospheric Deposition Program, National Trends Network, Retrieved from https://nadp.slh.wisc.edu/

Detoxification Organs

Detoxification Organs

It is very important to understand the organs involved in detoxification and how these systems work. The organs involved are the:
- Intestines
- Liver
- Skin
- Lungs
- Kidney
- Lymphatic Systems.

Defining Detoxification Organs
1. Digestive System- consists of many organs. The hollow organs make up most of the GI tract and consist of the mouth, esophagus, stomach, small intestine, large intestine, and colon. There are also solid organs such as the liver, pancreas, kidney, and gallbladder that are part of the digestive system.
    1.1. Small Intestine- the portion of the intestine that runs between the stomach and the large intestine; also sectioned as the duodenum (upper portion), jejunum (middle portion), and ileum (lower portion).
    1.2. Large Intestine- the large bowel is where water is absorbed, the remaining waste material is stored here as feces, feces is removed here by defecation, and the large bowel is the last part of the gastrointestinal tract in the digestive system.
    1.3. Colon- absorbs water and other nutrients not absorbed during small intestine and large intestine digestion.
2. Liver- a large lobed organ located in the abdomen, and it is involved in many metabolic processes.
    2.1. Gallbladder- the small sac-shaped organ beneath the liver, in which bile is stored after secretion by the liver and before release into the intestine.
3. Skin- a thin layer of tissue that forms the outer covering of the human body.
4. Lungs- a pair of organs that draws in air so that oxygen can pass into the blood and carbon dioxide can be removed from the blood.
5. Kidneys- a pair of organs working together in a unanimous fashion to filter out nitrates through urine.
6. Lymphatic System- a network of vessels through which lymph, a colorless fluid made to clean tissues, that drains from the tissues into the blood.

Organ systems are used in combination with the digestive tract and liver to help complete the detoxification processes. It takes a group effort to complete the process of detox, even though the liver does most of the work. If these organ systems are unable to function correctly, it will be difficult for the liver to complete its job.

Eating
After food is chewed, swallowed, and makes its way to the stomach, the pancreas organ releases pancreatic enzymes to help break down the food, the enzymes then help keep the small intestine in becoming free from harmful bacteria. If the pancreas isn't working sufficiently, then the risk of getting an intestinal infection is more significant.

Gastrointestinal
The digestive tract helps break down food and consumed liquids with the help of hydrochloric acid (HCL), bile from the gallbladder, and digestive enzymes from the pancreas. Intestinal cells have an efflux detox system that uses small amounts of phase 1 and phase 2 enzymes produced by the liver to help eliminate toxic load (Shimizu, 2012).

The small intestine is where the nutrients are absorbed. If this organ system becomes infected with pathogens, it cannot work correctly, and nutrients needed for physiological process and detoxification are minimized. If nutrients are minimal, the liver will struggle to convert the necessary nutrients needed to reduce free radicals in the bloodstream.

Liver
The liver is the body's largest endocrine gland. It has over 200 functions and can control carbohydrate, protein, fat, and steroid (cholesterol) metabolisms. The liver also breaks down red blood cells, synthesizes blood proteins, and regulates blood clotting factors. Additionally, it helps to convert nitrogenous compounds (amino acids) such as ammonia to urea (urine), helps to form and produce bile, and detoxifies the body of unwanted substances. Therefore, it's best if we make efforts to care for it enormously so it can carry out its functions.

Of all functions, the primary purpose of the liver is to filter and detoxify the blood. The blood can contain foreign invaders, antigen-antibody complexes, bacteria and viruses, and other toxins. The cells of the liver network are smart and can recognize these. Thus, the liver is so powerful and it can clear nearly 99% of these invaders in just the first cycle through it.

A major function of the liver is the responsibility of the elimination of drugs, alcohol, and xenobiotics while degrading hormones and synthesizing numerous varying molecules. It needs to be able to complete metabolic functions to add or remove amino groups from other molecules to create the reactions necessary to move free radicals through phase 1 and phase 2 detoxification processes.

As stated in the previous chapter, for the body to remove free radicals, the

Detoxification Organs

body uses water. The water is used to complete free radical orbit and in addition is used to remove these same toxins and other waste brought into our bodies. When the liver completes a filter cycle, the waste is either removed via urine by kidneys or through intestines via bile production from the liver and movement in the digestive tract.

Gallbladder and Bile

The bile is formed in the liver cells, then stored in the gallbladder. In particular, bile is a significant carrier of toxins. These toxins helps keep the small intestine pathogen-free. The toxins in bile also help break down fats and bind with fiber from food. During this process, the combination of bile and fiber are able to attract pathogens on it's way through the intestine. As the mixture moves down toward the colon, water and other nutrients are absorbed into the colon leaving behind the toxic residue. After binding with bile and fiber, this residue is released from the colon.

If you have no gallbladder, there can be some severe issues with the bile. While you still have bile produced from the liver going into your intestines, the body will not be able to routinely signal the gallbladder to release this bile. The release will be sporadic, and without a gallbladder, it's excreted as soon as liver makes it. The body needs routine signalling between the gallbladder and the liver for the release mechanisms of bile to function properly. Having your gallbladder removed can impair the body's ability to remove toxic compounds from ingested foods and food related pathogens, and this puts individuals at risk for nutrient deficiencies leading to disease.

Fact:
People with no gallbladder or poor bile health can't break down fats properly. When eating fatty foods, the fats remain intact, running through the intestinal system. This leads to smelly and runny stools.

Skin
The major function of the skin is to remove waste products, toxicants, and excess micronutrients by the process of sweating and preventing toxin entry by acting as a barrier (Baker, 2019).

Lungs
The major function of the lungs is to absorb oxygen. Although oxygen is needed to survive, it still becomes a toxin through the process of cellular respiration (IH, 2016). Cellular respiration is the process in which cells convert consumed energy into chemical energy (aka ATP) (IH, 2016). Oxygen is needed for this process to be completed. However, during this process an end product called "carbon dioxide" is produced (IH, 2016). Lungs are needed to make the exchange between oxygen and carbon dioxide.

Thus, they detox the body of carbon dioxide.

Kidneys

The kidneys are a "pair" of organs that assist in the removal of toxins form the blood (Ogobuiro & Tuma, 2022). They produce urine to remove the toxins from the body and transfer them to the genitals for excretion (Ogobuiro & Tuma, 2022). Also, other functions of the kidneys are to control osmolarity (how concentrated the blood is), help facilitate electrolyte balance by keeping a sodium and potassium ratio well distributed, and ensure vitamin D conversion is complete (Ogobuiro & Tuma, 2022). Additionally, if the kidneys aren't functioning correctly, then waste created from nitrogenous compounds cannot efficiently be removed via urea cycle.

Lymphatic System

The major function of the lymphatic system is to use the immune system to help eliminate xenobiotics, neutralize harmful substances that come from the environment, and eliminate harmful pathogens or byproducts that come from diseased cells (IH, 2020).

Phases of Detoxification

Phases of Detoxification

Nutrients play pivotal roles in the two distinct phases of liver detoxification, commonly referred to as Phase 1 and Phase 2 detoxification. *Phase 1,* known as Cytochrome P450 Enzymes, initiates the process, while *Phase 2,* termed Conjugated Pathways, continues the transformation (Phang-Lyn & Llerena, 2021). At times, one phase might function optimally while the other lags behind. Alternatively, neither phase could be operating efficiently. Furthermore, even when both phases are on track, insufficient availability of required nutrients and cofactors can hinder their performance. FInally, *phase3,* recognized as Elimination, is the final step in this intricate process (Phang-Lyn & Llerena, 2021).

Each phase relies on a distinct selection of nutrients, enzymes, and cofactors to execute their specific tasks.

- *Phase 1* designated nutrients facilitate the breakdown of chemicals and toxins, transforming them into metabolites suitable for further metabolism.
- *Phase 2* follows by taking these newly formed metabolites and proceeding with their metabolization.

What is Detoxification?
Detoxification is the process of the liver converting <u>non-polar, lipid soluble</u> molecules into <u>polar, water soluble molecules</u> (Phang-Lyn & Llerena, 2021).

Figure 3: *Phases of Detoxification*

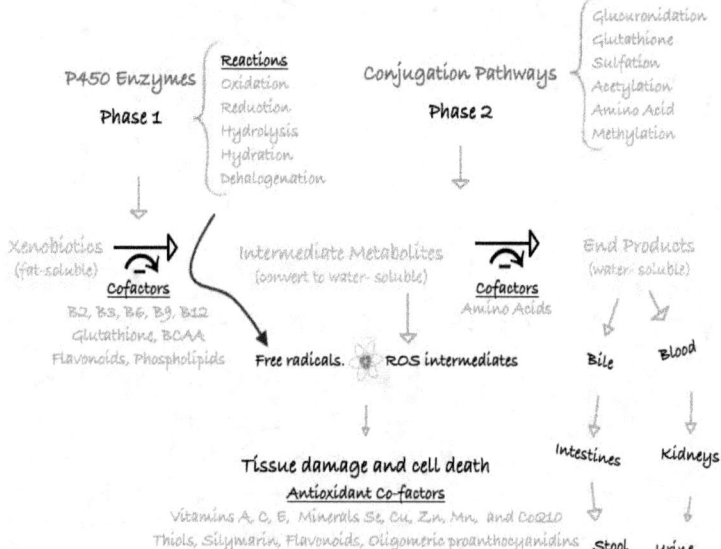

During phase 1 of detoxification,, the liver employs the P450 cytochrome enzymes to modify molecules by introducing oxygen, water, or halogens, or by reducing oxygen, water, or halogens from the molecule (Phang-Lyn & Llerena, 2021). These reactions are termed oxidation, hydrolysis, hydration, dehalogenation, or reduction (Phang-Lyn & Llerena, 2021). Consequently, the molecule undergoes transformations and becomes an intermediate byproduct commonly recognized as a free radical!

Following this, the resultant byproducts progress into phase 2 detoxification (Phang-Lyn & Llerena, 2021). During this stage, conjugates continue the process by converting the toxins into a polar, water soluble molecules (Phang-Lyn & Llerena, 2021). Phase 2 facilitates this conversion by introducing additional molecular groups to the free radical molecules. This alteration further reduces toxins, rendering them more water-soluble and thereby enabling their elimination from the body (Phang-Lyn & Llerena, 2021).

Phase 1
In Phase 1 of detoxification, a key nutrient utilized is *reduced nicotinamide adenine dinucleotide phosphate hydroge*n (NADPH), along with oxygen to carry out its functions (Phang-Lyn & Llerena, 2021). As free radicals combine with water and transform into superoxides, they can be converted into substances that can be filtered through the kidneys. Subsequently, the body eliminates them through urine.

The cytochrome P450 enzymes are chiefly responsible for eliminating xenobiotics and external toxins from the body (Phang-Lyn & Llerena, 2021). This pathway is notably involved in detoxifying substances such as anticonvulsants, antidepressants, sedatives, narcotics, antibiotics, anticoagulants, analgesics, steroids, antihistamines, tranquilizers, and more (Phang-Lyn & Llerena, 2021). Moreover, Phase 1 contributes to detoxifying commonly used over-the-counter medications like aspirin and salicylic acids, as well as food toxins like caffeine and alcohol. It is also involved in processing environmental toxins such as cigarette smoke, vehicle exhaust, paint fumes, pesticides, perfumes, and chemicals from personal care products.

When activated, Phase 1 aims to neutralize these toxins. However, inhibitors can hinder Phase 1 from breaking down toxins, allowing them to circulate in the bloodstream for an extended period, which can be detrimental. This situation can sometimes be referred to as an overdose, where an excessive amount of toxic substances is present in the blood. Overdoses can stem from various sources, including food, chemicals, drugs, or products.

Phases of Detoxification

- **Inhibitors'** impact on the Phase 1 detoxification include antihistamines, tranquilizers, stomach acid blocking drugs, bacterial and fungi fighting drugs, and specific phytonutrients such as naringenin from grapefruit juice (Phang-Lyn & Llerena, 2021), quercetin from onions, curcumin, and capsaicin.
- **Inducers** of Phase 1 detoxification can be drugs, air pollutants, alcohol,, cigarette smoke, pesticides, charcoal-grilled meats, high protein diets, saturated fats, indoles from cruciferous vegetables (Phang-Lyn & Llerena, 2021).

Phase 1 can be influenced by genetics, nutrient status, and toxin exposure. If the toxins are not eliminated via kidneys, then they move on to Phase 2.

Phase 2
Primary pathways Phase 2 detoxification employs several primary pathways, including glutathione conjugation (unification), amino acid conjugation, methylation, sulfation, acetylation, and glucuronidation to complete its operations (Phang-Lyn & Llerena, 2021). The specific pathway chosen depends on the type of toxin present in the body and the optimal method for for its elimination. The selection of nutrients for Phase 2 detoxification can vary depending on the toxins and the pathways being utilized, allowing for a diverse range of nutrient combinations.

Phase 2 pathways are essential for removing medications, drugs, and xenobiotics (Phang-Lyn & Llerena, 2021), and internal compounds such as recycled vitamins, minerals, amino acids, steroids, and hormones that are no longer needed. Additionally, Phase 2 is responsible for eliminating external compounds obtained from foods and beverages. Most importantly, Phase 2 plays a crucial role in the elimination of free radicals, contributing to overall detoxification processes.

Inhibitors of Phase 2 can hinder the breakdown of toxins, leading to the accumulation of extremely harmful toxins within the body. Since free radicals are formed after Phase 1, some toxins are converted into dangerous compounds, as specific reactions are necessary to facilitate their mixing with bile, aiding in the removal of harmful toxins and pathogens (Phang-Lyn & Llerena, 2021).

- **Inhibitors'** impact on the Phase 2 pathways varies on the pathway being utilized.
    - Deficiencies in selenium, glutathione, and zinc can affect glutathione conjugation.
    - Low protein diets can affect amino acid conjugation.
    - Deficiencies in vitamins B2, B3, B6, folic acid or vitamin B12 can

Phases of Detoxification

   impact methylation.
    - NSAIDs (non-steroidal anti-inflammatory drugs) such as aspirin, a deficiency in molybdenum, and food colorings like yellow food dye can affect sulphation.
    - Deficiencies in Vitamin B2, B5, or C can impact acetylation.
    - Drugs that eliminate uric acid or NSAIDs can influence glucuronidation.
- **Inducers** of Phase 2 detoxification also varies with the pathway being utilized for detoxification.
    - The amino acid glycine can affect amino acid conjugation.
    - Amino acids cysteine, methionine, taurine impact sulphation.
    - Goitrogenic foods from the Brassica family can influence glutathione conjugation.
    - Fish oil and birth control pills, or steroidal hormones can affect glucuronidation.
    - So far, there has been no research that has found an inducer of the acetylation pathway in regards to ridding the body of toxins. However, B5 supports the path. Therefore, if someone lacks B5, this pathway will have difficulties with detoxing methods.
    - Just as folic acid and vitamin B12 inhibits methylation, methylation is also induced them, along with the amino acid methionine.

Balancing Phase 1 and Phase 2 detoxification is crucial, as the equilibrium between these phases is necessary to prevalent the circulation of free radicals in the human body. Imbalances can lead to Phase 1 intolerance to certain toxins, making it more challenging to eliminate these substances. Thus, their conversion rates must be aligned, Phase 1's rate of converting toxins into other compounds to be eliminated should match Phase 2's ability to take over and perform its role.

Antioxidants

What are antioxidants?

Antioxidants are compounds that play a vital role in preventing or slowing down damage to cells caused by free radicals or unstable molecules. These substances work to inhibit oxidation by initiating specific signals that guide the assembly and delivery of suitable antioxidants to remove harmful free radicals (Al-Mamary & Moussa, 2021). This process involves the donation of an electron or hydrogen free radical to effectively scavenge other free radicals seeking to form damaging pairs (Al-Mamary & Moussa, 2021).

Antioxidants that have donating capabilities are:
- Ascorbic acid (vitamin C)
- Uric acid
- Glutathione
- Tocopherols (vitamin E)
- Polyhydroxy phenolic compounds (found in plants)

Antioxidant enzymes prevent toxic substances from accumulating and destroying tissues. They repair DNA enzymes including polymerases, glycosylases and nucleases and proteolytic enzymes such as proteinases, proteases and peptidases located in the cytosol and mitochondria (Al-Mamary & Moussa, 2021). Antioxidant are well renowned for their ability to counteract oxidative stress, a phenomenon that significantly contributes to the prevention of diseases with fatal outcomes.

Major antioxidant enzymes that suppress free radicals and ROS are:
- Superoxide dismutase (SOD)
- Catalase (CAT)
- Glutathione peroxidase (GPx)

The Remarkable Benefits of Plant Life

The intrinsic properties of plants hold the potential to enhance longevity, as scientists have found the phenolic compounds present in plants contribute significantly to the reversal and prevention of various diseases.

Key Role in Primary Energy Dynamics

Undoubtedly, the sun stands as the predominant energy source on our planet, with plants and algae directly harnessing its energy. Through this process, plants synthesize their own essential nutrients, facilitating their survival. Thus, plants emerge as the foundational wellspring of energy for all terrestrial ecosystems.

The highest productivity of plants is observed in regions characterized by warmth, humidity, and ample sunlight, which collectively foster optimal conditions for their growth and energy absorption.

Food Chain: Ecological Food Relationships

Within the intricate tapestry of ecosystems, species that derive food from plants are considered primary consumers or herbivores. This group encompasses animals, insects, and even humans, often referred to as vegetarians. Primary consumers, who get their direct consumption of plant matter, access primary energy, which is attributed to the rich nutrient content of plants.

Conversely, secondary energy, derived from the consumption (the eating) of primary consumers like animals and insects, is relatively less efficient. This category involves carnivores or meat-eaters. Secondary consumers extract comparatively lower energy from their diet, as much of the energy obtained by primary consumers has already been expended for their bodily functions.

However, the reduced energy efficiency of secondary consumers carries potential risks. Primary consumers tend to ingest toxins in minimal quantities, which they then metabolically transform into biological toxins, subsequently stored within their bodies until detoxification is feasible. Given this accumulation, the concentration of toxins intensifies. When secondary consumers consume primary consumers, they inadvertently ingest these toxins as well. While plant consumption is associated with increased human longevity, various factors contribute to this phenomenon, as outlined below.

Nutrient Conversion

The journey of converting nutrients from plants within the body involves a series of intricate processes. Nutrients derived from plants undergo this transformation before they become accessible for nourishment.

First nutrients are eaten, then they are converted when they need to be used. What doesn't need to be used will continue to circulate through the system and eliminated. Plant nutrients (primary energy sources) are easy to dispose of because if they haven't been converted for use they are still in their insoluble form. This makes it easier to digest and eliminate form the body.

Soluble nutrients, already converted sources from meats (secondary energy sources), are absorbed naturally and if not used will remain in circulation or stored until they can be detoxified and eliminated. After plants are converted this also occur for these nutrients.

Plant Antioxidants

Plants are natural sources of antioxidants and contain hydroxyl groups. Below is a list of plant antioxidants.

- Phenols have been documented to prevent cancer. Phenols include phenol, catechol, resorcinol, phloroglucinol, hydroquinone, and

pyrogallol.
- Phenolic acids such as hydroxybenzoic and hydroxycinnamic acids including benzoic acid, salicylic acid, gallic acid, syringic acid, vanillic acid, gentisic acid, protocatechuic acid, cinnamic acid, coumaric acid, ferulic acid, caffeic acid, and sinapic acid.
  Flavonoids are secondary metabolites and include green tea, black tea, coffee, vegetables, fruits, olive oil, wine made from grapes, and chocolate.
- Cyanidin and quercetin. Quercetin is found in onions, green tea, apples, berries and other plant foods.
- Stilbenes are related to polyphenols and include stilbene, resveratrol, piceatannol, and pterostilbene. Found in grapes, peanuts, and berries.

Chelating Nutrients
Iron, copper, and vitamin C are cofactors to antioxidant enzymes and should be eaten in combination with phenolic compounds. Phenolic compounds have chelating activity and helps reduce free radical formation. Since iron forms highly reactive oxides in the gut, it must be reduced from it's non-heme form (Fe^{3+}) to its heme form (Fe^{2+}) to ensure optimal utilization. Vitamin C forms a chelate with non-heme iron from plants and turns it into an absorbable form of heme-iron. Therefore, using the heme-iron from, which has polyhydroxylated properties, can help reduce hydroxyl free radical ions and contribute to cellular protection (Al-Mamary & Moussa, 2021).

People who eat more plants live longer!
Phenolic compounds from plants are core phytochemicals with health promoting properties (Swallah et al., 2020). Inadequate intake of phytonutrients results in the risk of certain diseases (Swallah et al., 2020). Phytonutrients are powerful antioxidants available in fruits and vegetables, but are richer in fruits (Swallah et al., 2020). Those that choose to not include healthy fruits and vegetables into their diet, have morbid consequences. Below is a list of fruits with the highest phenolics (Swallah et al., 2020).

Fruit	%mg
Lemons	843
Limes	751
Grapes	893
Blueberries	327
Raspberry black	670
Raspberry red	342
Raspberry yellow	426

Nutrients

Nutrients

Nutrients are classified as compounds that help boost physiological functions. They help improve energy, metabolism, body heat, cellular repair, and cellular growth. Most importantly, they help with detoxification processes. Vitamins, minerals, amino acids, hormones, and other nutrients have special roles they play in anti-oxidizing the body.

Detoxification involves a wide array of nutrients, and delving into the detailed biochemical properties of each would require a comprehensive book. As a result, we'll provide a list of the key nutrients participating in phase 1 and phase 2 processes, focusing on a select few for discussion.

Phase 1 Nutrients, Enzymes, and Cofactors
- Vitamin B2
- Vitamin B3
- Vitamin B6
- Folic Acid (B9)
- Vitamin B12
- Glutathione
- Branched Chain Amino Acids (BCAAs)
- Phenols (flavonoids from plants)
- Phospholipids

Antioxidants for Tissue Damage and Cell Death
Hydrophilic
- Thiols
- Ascorbic acid (vitamin C)
- Minerals such as selenium, copper, zinc, manganese
- Silymarin
- Phenols (flavonoids from plants)
- Oligomeric proanthocyanidins
- Glutathione

Lipophilic
- Beta Carotene (vitamin A)
- Ubiquinol (CoQ10)
- Tocopherols (vitamin E)

Phase 2 Nutrients, Enzymes, and Cofactors
- Glutathione
- Glucuronide
- Sulfur
- Acetyl-CoA
- Methyltransferases
- Amino Acids

Tocopherols (vitamin E)
Vitamin E protects polyunsaturated fatty acids (PUFA's), by preventing lipid oxidation. Vitamin E stops ROS when fat begins to undergo oxidation reactions. A popular subject around vitamin E is the reduction of low density lipoproteins (LDL) (high amounts of LDL cholesterol). In addition to its anti-oxidizing properties, it is known as an angiogenic type vitamin, the formation of new blood vessels, and anti-inflammatory vitamin for the reduction of inflammation.

There are many different forms of tocopherol including alpha, beta, delta, and gamma forms. All different forms of tocopherol are taken in by the liver and transformed into vitamin E. Alpha tocopherols accumulate in non-hepatic tissues such as the heart due to free radical production being extremely favored in these organs. Since mixed tocopherols work better together than separately, in combination they provide the antioxidant activity needed to fight free radical generation.

Vitamin E can be easily depleted by the extensive accumulation of free radicals as a result of constant consumption of toxic substances (ie. toxins coming from alcohol, cigarettes, chemically created sugars and diet sweeteners, or extreme exercise).

The richest food source for vitamin E are almonds, hazel nuts, sunflower seeds, green leafy vegetables, dark leafy greens, wheat germ, wheat germ oil, safflower oil, and sunflower oil, and other vegetable oils.

The recommended dietary allowance (RDA) for vitamin E for adults age 19 years and older is 15 mg per day or 22.4 IU international units. This is the average daily level of intake to meet sufficient requirements of nearly all healthy people (98%).

Ascorbic Acid (vitamin C)
Vitamin C is a proven antioxidant. This is because it reduces pro-oxidants. It also helps to preserve stores of vitamin E. In replenishing vitamin E, it donates electrons to regenerate vitamin E's lipid soluble antioxidant effects. In addition, niacin (B3) and thiols can regenerate Vitamin C.

This vitamin prevents, protects, improves, and controls a number of reactions in the body such as: immune function, protein oxidation, reduction of atherogenesis and LDL, improves elastin, produces collagen, improves tyrosine metabolism, and helps maintain healthy connective tissue.

Vitamin C is positively charged. It helps other nutrients accept hydrogen atoms from water and plays an important role in both phase 1 and phase 2 detoxification. Vitamin C also donates to at least 17 known enzymes in fungi,

Nutrients

pyrimidines, and components of DNA. In addition, vitamin C also donates to 14 other known enzymes that are single and double bound units of oxygen and hydrogen, that are utilized as antioxidants.

Vitamin C in foods can be depleted the longer a person preserves the food or even so, by cooking the food. So, vitamin C type foods are best eaten fresh or steamed. It is naturally found in fruits and vegetables. The richest food sources for vitamin C or ascorbic acid are strawberries, papayas, red bell peppers, kiwi, oranges, tomatoes, cantaloupe, broccoli, brussel sprouts, kale, snow peas, mangoes, fresh grapefruit, honey dew melon, mustard greens, cauliflower, tangerines, cabbage, sweet potatoes, potatoes, tomatoes, watermelons, and asparagus.

The RDA for healthy adults over the age of 19 years is a minimum of 90 mg per day for men and 75 mg per day for women.

B Vitamins and Methylation
B vitamins are important and are a family of vitamins that improve energy expenditure. These energy promoting vitamins help the synthesis of cholesterol and fatty acids along with other bodily functions. B vitamins, are well known for helping convert toxins to free radicals, but are also important for eliminating free radicals in support of methylation.

Methylation is used in both phase and phase 2 detoxification processes, and serves two major functions. One function is the transfer of methyl group N5-methyl-FH4 to homocysteine. If this does not happen a deficiency of vitamin B12 occurs, causing carbons to become trapped in the methyl form. The second function is the turnover of methylmalonyl CoA to succinyl CoA, which is required for conversion of "odd chain fatty acids."

The modification of toxins and chemicals occurs during phase 2 and clears the body of toxins. These toxins can be endogenous or external. Such toxins can alter methylation processes.

Phase 2 uses B1, B2, B3, B5, B6, B9, B12, and SAMe during methylation cycles, This is because B vitamins are key factors in the biochemical functions of methylation. During the methylation cycle, a methyl group is added to DNA molecules. Also as the methylation cycle continues, cofactors such as B2, B3, B6, folic acid, and B12 are necessary to complete the recycling of more methylation groups.

Methylation is like an on/off switch. Genes and molecules alike can be turned on or off by methylation. This occurs by transferring one methyl group to another. When detoxing toxins some methyl groups are added, while other groups are separated and removed.

B12: Cobalamin
Vitamin B12 is also known as Cobalamin. This popular vitamin cannot be synthesized by plants or animals. This is why vitamin B12 is the most crucial of all vitamins and minerals. It's role in detoxification is to maintain methylation balance with vitamin B9 (folate). Methylation is also the key to glutathione production. It helps by ridding the body of free radicals, especially heavy metals and carcinogens.

This rare vitamin can only be obtained from 2 food sources, dried green and purple algae. Yet, it can be sourced from animal products only after the animal has consumed bacteria. Fish, shellfish, meats, eggs, and dairy products can all be great sources of B12. But the highest source of meat to have vitamin B12 are those that natural eat bacteria in the wild.

The RDA is crucial for knowing if how much of this vitamin you may need to take. The RDA for adults 2.4 ug/d.

Depletions in any of the B vitamins can interfere with one-carbon metabolism. Thus, this can interfere with detoxification and other very important bodily functions.

A B-complex vitamin is a great way to get B vitamins. Nonetheless, eating meat or symbiotic plant/bacterial species such as seaweeds, as well as grains, herbs and other plant life are other great sources to acquire a variety of B vitamins.

Glutathione
Glutathione peroxidase is an antioxidant enzyme that needs minerals like selenium, copper, zinc and iron to function properly. It also interacts with vitamin E for proper lipid oxidation. Glutathione, is a naturally occurring antioxidant often found in all life, and is made from three amino acids glycine, cysteine, and glutamic acid.

Its role is to act as an antioxidant and rid the body of free radicals in preventing damage to cells caused by ROS. Glutathione directly neutralizes singlet oxygen species, hydroxyl radicals, and superoxide radicals. Additionally, it is known to help remove heavy metals such as mercury, help in mitochondrial function, aid in lipid peroxidation, and help repair, rebuild, and remove cells.

Glutathione has critical roles in detoxification. First, it acts as a cofactor for several antioxidant enzymes. Second, it aids in the regeneration of both vitamins C and E. Third, it plays a role in neutralizing of free radicals produced by Phase 1 detoxification by unifying the reactions of Phase 1 detox with hydrogens to make them easier to dispose of through the kidneys.

Glutathione also heals the gut by providing a direct fuel source for gastrointestinal cells. It neutralizes and oxidizes the gut lining almost instantly upon interaction. It also helps break down the byproducts created during digestion, increases absorption of the intestinal barrier, and aids in strengthening immune function in the gut.

Depletions can take a toll on red blood cells, while deficiency can be detrimental to detoxification processes.

Getting adequate glutathione from foods still help reduce disease state and improve detoxification processes. Foods with the highest content of glutathione are sulfur type foods including bone broth, meats, poultry, fish, shellfish, beans, onion family (onions, garlic, leeks, shallots, chives, etc...) and the cabbage family (brussels, broccoli, cabbage, kale, asparagus, cauliflower, and mustard greens, etc..). There is no RDA for glutathione. There have been no reported harmful side effects, therefore there is no upper limit (UL), which is the maximum we can take.

Selenium
Selenium is a very important mineral in the regulation of enzymes that are dependent on selenium to function properly. Such enzymes are glutathione peroxidase; thioredoxin reductase; iodothyronine deiodinases; selenoproteins P, W, V, and S; selenophosphate synthetase, methionine, and sulfoxide reductases. These enzymes are imperative for regeneration of antioxidants, and play a role in phase 1 and phase 2 detoxification processes.

Selenium actually will protect against oxidative stress in the body because the glutathione protein is a selenoprotein and needs selenium for creation. As selenoproteins aid in the reduction of carcinogen type cells that are created due to overload of toxins.

Deficiency of selenium is not uncommon and can lead to decreased activity of the enzymes listed above. This is because it does so much to detoxify the body, it gets depleted so easily. With vitamin E deficit selenium will decrease to try a make up for detoxification processes.

Foods richest in selenium are any type of fish especially cod fish, yellowfin tuna, liver, ground beef, turkey meat, spinach, salmon, trout, sardines, flounder, halibut, shrimp, lobster, oysters, chicken breasts, brazil nuts, cashews, lentils, brown rice, and other nuts, mushrooms, and shellfish.

The RDA is imperative to know because if we are too low or too high in selenium then we can figure out how much we should be taking. The RDA the average adult 19 yrs and older is 55 mcg/d and the upper limit (UL), which is the maximum amount we can take, is 400 mcg/d.

Nutrients

Milk Thistle in Modern Holistic's

Silymarin also known as milk thistle, in modern holistic's, lowers cholesterol, enhances liver function, and improves diabetes!

Hepatics are used in herbal medicine to cleanse the liver, and strengthen the flow of bile in the gallbladder. Bitters (herbs or plants that predominantly have a bitter taste) and Cholagogues (help secrete bile fluids) are both hepatics, and both aid in the improvement of gastrointestinal organ function and digestion. Milk Thistle is a hepatic and galactagogue (helps release milk or flow of other fluids), and has alkalizing properties, bitters properties, and cholagogue properties. Alkaloids are nitrogen containing herbs and vegetables which help balance fluid flow. Milk Thistle can protect the liver against toxins, which in turn allow for the liver to deliver substantial results.

In modern holistic medicine, many of the old and all of the new practitioners use a complementary and alternative approach to healing and treating diseases. This includes the use of herbs as medicine instead of conventional techniques that utilize genetically engineered pharmaceutical pills. Integrative practitioners use both conventional and complementary techniques.

Nutritional Methods

Nutritional Methods

Medical Nutrition Therapy
Nutritional diagnostics, therapies, and counseling services are conducted for the purpose of disease management. These services are completed by a registered dietitian (RD) or a nutrition professional called a certified nutrition specialist (CNS). An RD can hold a bachelor's, master's, or doctoral degree and a CNS can only hold a master's or doctoral degree. Both of these professionals can be licensed in their state of residence and the license identification is Licensed Dietitian Nutritionist (LDN).

Medical Nutrition Therapy (MNT) is a specific application of a process we call the Nutrition Care Process. It provides a focus of the management of diseases in clinical settings through a nutritional approach. MNT involves in-depth individualized nutrition assessment, nutritional therapy, and nutritional counseling. Throughout a person's recovery or management of a disease state, a LDN will be there to guide them through. In other words, for nutrition support and management of a medical diagnosis, MNT can help an individual learn the lifestyle and dietary strategies to manage these medical challenges.

Many diseases require the process of detoxification. This is one of the strategies nutritionists will focus on. Also, flushing of toxins or system repair will require vitamins and minerals, and other holistic practices. This is to aid in the detoxing process because most diseases are caused by some deficit or excess of micronutrients.

Detoxification Questionnaires
First, a person cannot detox without first going through a series of health questionnaires. The first questionnaire is a thorough health application that reviews medical history, family history, lifestyle, sleep cycles, medication and nutraceutical usage, lab findings, and other very important factors. Other questionnaires can be completed prior to seeing a nutrition specialist and these can be toxin questionnaires or other lifestyle questionnaires.

The following pages have toxin questionnaires that review environmental exposures; emotional, social, and spiritual life stressors; dietary patterns; xenobiotic tolerability; and a general wellness symptoms assessment.

Nutritional Methods

Detoxification Questionnaire

Environmental Exposures
Please read the following symptoms and circle yes or no.

Do any of these negatively affect you or do you develop symptoms upon exposure to:						
Dust	Y	N	Glues or sealants	Y	N
Perfume	Y	N	New car smell	Y	N
Animals	Y	N	Gasoline fumes	Y	N
Mold	Y	N	Grass, ragweed, or tree pollen	Y	N
Paints	Y	N	Fabric store	Y	N
Rubber	Y	N	Soaps/Detergents	Y	N
Cosmetics	Y	N	Air conditioner	Y	N
Hair spray	Y	N	Tobacco smoke	Y	N

Total number of yes's _____ Total number of no's _____

Do you use any of these or have any of these near you at home or work?						
Asphalt/Tar	Y	N	Chlorinated water/Water purifier	Y	N
Swamp	Y	N	Area rugs/Carpeting	Y	N
Damp cellar	Y	N	Wood/Coal stove	Y	N
Woods	Y	N	Gas appliances	Y	N
Moth ball	Y	N	Feather bedding/pillows	Y	N
Dump	Y	N	Kerosene space heater	Y	N
Chemicals	Y	N	Urea formaldehyde or insulation	Y	N
Electric blanket	Y	N	Pesticide treatments on house exterior	Y	N

Total number of yes's _____ Total number of no's _____
Total number of yes's from both tables _____ Total number of yes's from both tables _____

Emotional, Social, and Spiritual Life Stressors
Please read the following stressors and check which one you experience.

Check all that apply:			
Home		**Work**	
Change in residence		Work tension	
Foreclosure		Loss of job	
New Mortgage		Change in work responsibility	
Family		More than 40-hr work week	
Marital stress		Retirement	
Divorce		**Sleep**	
Marital separation or problems		Too little rest	
Teenage problem children		Change in sleep patterns	
Small children at home stressors		**Personal**	
Children leaving the house		Personal injury or illness	
Pregnancy stressors		Drug or alcohol addiction	
Child added to family (Step or foster children/ adoption)		Loss of self-confidence	
Family death		Trouble with law	
Change in health for family member		Difficulties with peers	
In-law challenges		Change in social activities	
Spiritual		Excessive worry	
Loss of meaning and purpose		Self defeating thoughts	
Lack of spiritual connection		Anger, guilt, fear, and hopelessness	
Disconnect from natural environments		Overstimulation of electronic devices	
No sense of belonging		Other _____	

Total number of check marks _____ Total number of blanks _____

Dietary Patterns
Please read the following and log points.

Log accordingly the number of times you do the following:	
1. Number of times you consume vegetables ☐ daily ☐ weekly (daily add 2 more pts)	
2. Number of times of you consume fruit ☐ daily ☐ weekly (daily add 2 more pts)	
3. Weekly number of times you consume meat	
4. Weekly number of times you consume whole grains	
5. Weekly number of times you consume nuts and seeds	
6. Weekly number of times you consume legumes	
7. Weekly number of times you consume small freshwater or ocean fish	
8. Daily number of times you consume water	
9. Weekly number of times you consume meat or bone broth	
10. Weekly number of times you purchase and eat fast food	
11. Weekly number of times you eat out at restaurants	
12. Daily number of times you consume dairy products	
13. Weekly number of times you consume sushi	
14. Weekly number of times you consume large deep ocean fish	
15. Number of times you consume high fructose corn syrup foods and beverages	
16. Daily number of time you consume caffeine or coffee	
17. Daily number of times you consume processed foods	
18. Daily number of times you consume trans-fats or saturated fats	
19. Number of times you consume alcohol ☐ daily ☐ weekly ☐ monthly (daily add 2 more pts)	
Total number of points for questions 1-9 _____ Total number of points for questions 10-19 _____	

Nutritional Methods 40

Xenobiotic Tolerability
Please answer the following and log points.

Check all that apply:		
Are you currently using prescription drugs? If yes, how many are you currently taking? ____ (ad 1 pt.extra for each medication)	Y	N
Are you currently taking one or more of the following OTC drugs? (add 2 pts extra for each one checked) ❏ Cimetidine ❏ Acetaminophen ❏ Estradiol	Y	N
If you have used or presently using prescription drugs, which of the following scenarios best represents your response to them:	Y	N
Experience side effects, the drug(s) is or are effective at lowered dose(s) (3 extra pts.)		
Experience side effects, the drug(s) is or are effective at usual dose(s) (2 extra pts.)		
Experience no side effects, the drug(s) is or are usually not effective (1 extra pt.)		
Experience no side effects, the drug(s) is or are usually effective (0 extra pt.)		
Are you currently taking any supplements?	Y	N
If so, what supplement (s)? _____ ❏ B-Complex ❏ Selenium ❏ Zinc ....(`1 pt for each box checked) ❏ Glutathione ❏ Vitamin C ❏ Vitamin E ❏ Amino acids (-2 pts for each box checked)		
Do you feel ill after you consume even small amounts of alcohol?	Y	N
Do you smoke, vape, or consume THC? ❏ Daily (2 pts extra) ❏ Weekly (1 pt extra) ❏ Monthly (0pt)	Y	N
Do you presently use or within the last 6 months have you regularly used tobacco products?	Y	N
Do you have strong negative reactions to tobacco or tobacco containing products?	Y	N
Do you have strong negative reactions to caffeine or caffeine containing products?	Y	N
Do you have an adverse or allergic reaction when you consume sulfite containing foods such as wine, dried fruit, salad bar vegetables, etc?	Y	N
Do you have a history of significant exposure to harmful chemicals such as herbicides, insecticides, pesticides, or organic solvents?	Y	N
Do you have an adverse or allergic reaction when you consume high histamine-containing foods such as wine, chocolate, cheese, orange juice, and bone broth?	Y	N
Do you have mercury fillings inside your mouth?	Y	N
Have you had long term exposure to arsenic, lead, lead paint, cadmium, cadmium-containing cigarettes, aluminum, or aluminum-containing deodorant such as aerosol deodorants?	Y	N
Have you had an antibiotic regimen within the last three months?	Y	N
Total number of yes's _____ No's _____ Extra points _____ Minus points _____		

General Wellness Symptoms Assessment

Please read the following and check which one you experience.

Check all that apply:

Liver/Gallbladder		Lungs	
Pain in the right shoulder blade		Post nasal drip	
Yellow, gray, white, or green stools		Chest congestion	
Foul smelly flatulence or stools		Shallow breathing	
Muscle aches		Itchy feet	
Kidney		**Mind/Brain**	
Dark circles under your eyes		Fatigue	
Puffy eyes		Depression or anxiety	
Lower back pain		Brain fog	
Dark urine		Mood swings	
Urine odor		Sleep interruptions or poor sleep duration	
Gastrointestinal System		**Skin**	
Nausea		Rashes	
Excessive burping after meals or drinks		Keratin build up	
Diarrhea		Red dots on your legs	
Constipation		Dry itchy or scaly skin	
Bloating after eating or drinking		Excessive sweating	
Heartburn		Flushing or hot flashes	
Facial acne		Aging or wrinkles	
Frequent headaches		Adverse body odor	
Circulatory		**Lymphatic System**	
Pain in your left arm		Persistent infections	
Chest pain		Recurrent colds	
Rapid or irregular heart beat		Frequent illness	

Total number of check marks _____ Total number of blanks _____

Nutritional Methods

Scoring Tool

Check all that apply:

Environmental Exposure		Dietary Patterns	
Total number of yes's		Total number of questions 1-9	
Total number of no's		Total number of questions 10-19	
If you scored more than 18 points in yes's, your environmental exposure to toxins is significant and exposure reduction methods is recommended.		If you scored more than 10 points on questions 10-19 then your exposure to dietary toxins is significant and exposure reduction is recommended.	
Emotional, Social, and Spiritual		General Wellness	
Total number of checks		Total number of checks	
Total number of blanks		Total number of blanks	
If you scored more than 18 points in checks, you have significant exposure to emotional stress and utilizing stress management techniques is recommended		If you scored more than 20 points in checks, you have significant metabolic toxin exposure and a detoxification plan is recommended.	
Liver/gallbladder detox more than 2 points, kidney detox more than 3 points, mind/brain system more than 3 points, gastrointestinal system detox more than 4 points, lungs more than 2 points, skin detox more than 4 points, and circulatory or lymphatic systems detox more than 1 points,			
Xenobiotic Tolerability		Detoxification Protocols	
Total number of yes's		Environmental Detox	
Total number of no's		Emotional, Social, and Spiritual Detox	
Extra points		Dietary Detox	
Minus points		General Wellness Detox	
If you scored more than 10 points, you have low xenobiotic tolerability and managing detoxification effectively and regularly is recommended.		Xenobiotic Detox	
Add number of yes's, number of check marks and extra points.			
Add number of no's, blanks and minus points.			
Subtract the second line from the first line.			
Total			
If you scored more than 76 points, it is highly recommended to try all 5 detoxification protocols.			

How do we detox?

How do we detox?   44

Eating Healthy is Ignored in Society
Consuming the appropriate foods plays a crucial role in promoting longevity, as these foods provide our bodies with the necessary nutrients. Unfortunately, many individuals do not maintain a well-balanced diet, which can elevate the risk of diseases. While doctors often suggest that supplementation is only needed for specific deficiencies in vitamins or minerals, this assumes that the average person is already following a nutritious diet.

Interesting Insight: Despite approximately 95% of family physicians endorsing the importance of healthy eating and lifestyle, fewer than 12% actually discuss these topics with their patients, and less than 6% incorporate them into their prescriptions.

Who will benefit form a detoxification protocol?
- Individuals exposed to trauma or continued excessive stress.
- People who have autoimmune disease diagnoses or systemic inflammation disorders.
- People who have metabolic diagnoses such as cardiovascular disease, thyroid disease, hyperlipidemia, diabetes, or insulin dysregulation disorders.
- Individuals highly susceptible to gaining weight.
- People who have alcohol use or substance use disorders, or chemical dependencies to foods, beverages, sugars, or caffeine.
- People who have diagnoses of mental health conditions or GI disorders.
- Individuals exposed daily to chemicals or heavy metals daily.

Removing toxic substances helps enhance the body's organs ability to absorb nutrients and its ability to use these nutrients for improved cellular function. Ultimately, it improves the healing process, and we can live longer and happier lives.

Examples of ways to detox are:
- Avoiding all proinflammatory foods
- Engaging in exercise
- Reducing stress
- Focusing on high quality macro and micro nutrients
- Eating foods to support liver and kidney organs
- Increasing antioxidant intake
- Using organic or plant based skin treatments
- Increasing water intake

The Program
The Program True Paleo Inc has developed a range of detox-friendly meal plans that not only support the detoxification process but also meet the minimum recommended dietary allowances. This guide provides you with various tools to ensure accurate and straightforward recipe preparation and meal planning.

Helpful Tip: Before embarking on any dietary protocol, it's advisable to consult the RDA provided by the US government for your specific age group and gender.

Maintaining Regular Eating Habits
Throughout the detox period, you'll continue to eat as you normally would. This means no skipping meals. If your usual routine involves three meals a day, you'll stick to that pattern. And if you typically eat three meals but still feel hungry, you're free to consume the necessary amount to satisfy your body's needs. Calorie counting and restrictive measures aren't part of this meal plan. Additionally, your meal timing preferences—whether you eat immediately upon waking or later in the day—remain unchanged.

Smart Shopping
A helpful shopping approach is to wait until your refrigerator and pantry are devoid of toxic foods before heading to the store. Purchase all your ingredients in one go, and then set aside time to prepare everything for the entire week. This way, you won't need to juggle cooking while focusing on detoxing.

Plan Ahead
Create a well-structured timeline that accommodates shopping, recipe preparation, and logging. As you plan your meals, take the opportunity to cultivate a mindful connection with your food. This will enable you to conduct an insightful "self assessment" of your emotional and physical responses. These practices will facilitate your progress and enhance open communication with your nutritionist and physician.

Grocery Store Tips & Tads
Recommended Store: *Whole Foods (not endorsed)*
- When shopping at the grocery store, it is good practice to ensure you purchase your veggies in their freshest state.
- Confirm that the veggies are 100% organic and are marked with the USDA stamp on the packaging. Organic means:
    - Food that has been farmed or produced without adding chemicals, pesticides, or artificial fertilizers to plants.
    - Meats are produced without adding hormones into animals tissues.
- Grass-fed and range free means:
    - Animals are not locked up in tiny cages, that they are free to roam around eating the grass and other live plants of the earth.

How do we detox?

- Also, ensure that the veggies DNA has not been genetically modified through genetic engineering.
- In addition, the veggies you choose should not be overly ripe, nor should they not be ripe enough.
- Ensure your veggies are vibrant in color. This reason is so that their phytonutrient content can act as stronger antioxidants.
    - Avoid yellowing leaves and vegetables with browning spots.
    - Herbs should be bought fresh.
    - Dried herbs can be substituted.

Shopping List
Vegetables
- Jerusalem artichokes, cabbage (large head), dandelion greens, collard greens, peas, carrots, red bell pepper, celery stalk, purple onion, and garlic cloves

Herbs
- Basil, cilantro, dill weed, oregano, parsley, rosemary, sage, thyme, cumin, and ground sea salt *Meats*
- Chicken legs or thighs, beef rib tips, pork ribs, shrimp, fish, organic sausage, beef chunks, and lamb chops.

Other
- Honey, ginger root, lemons, dried agar seaweed, brazil nuts, sunflower seeds (unsalted), Haas avocado (black), strawberries, blueberries

Supplements (not endorsed)
- Nutra Pro, Virgin Cod Liver Oil, Pure Encapsulations, Ascorbic Acid: for a more cost effective option choose Now vitamins.

Eliminate Sensitivities
There are 14 food allergens that are recognized across the globe. In America, the Food and Drug Administration (FDA) and the US Department of Agriculture (USDA) only recognizes 8 food allergens to specific proteins. In Europe the Food Information Regulation (FIR) and the Food Information for Consumers Regulation (FICR) recognize 14 food allergens to specific proteins. The next 2 pages cover cover these 14 food allergens, other possible names they could go by, and list ways that these foods could be served or packaged. If you experience any sensitivities to any of these foods groups please refer to the correct list for removal from your diet.

1. Fish- anchovies, bass, catfish, cod, flounder, grouper, haddock, halibut, herring, Mahi Mahi, swordfish, perch, pike, pollock, red fish, salmon, sole, or snapper, tilapia, trout, or tuna.
2. Soy- flours or powders, soy milks or curds, soy formulas, miso, soy

How do we detox?

   beans or pods, soy protein, soy pulp, tempeh or tofu, edamame, soy sprouts, soy albumins or soy fiber; soy butters, oils, or sauces; soy seasons or substitutes.
3. **Crustaceans**- crabs, Hermit Crabs, crayfish, lobsters, mantis, prawns or shrimp, or sea spiders.
4. **Eggs**- egg albumin or ovalbumin, cholesterol free eggs, cage free eggs, organic eggs, dried eggs or powder, egg white, egg yolk, eggnog, meringue, mayonnaise, or egg wash.
5. **Peanuts**- ground or seeds, peanut flours or powders; peanut butters, oils, or sauces; peanut paste or nut meat, peanut extract, peanut protein, peanuts boiled or cold pressed, peanuts extruded or expelled, or peanut syrup.
6. **Mollusks**- oysters, clams or cockles, snails or conch, squid or octopus, scallops, or mussels.
7. Sulfur-oxides- dried fruits, dried vegetables, soft drinks, alcoholic beverages, sulphur, sulphur dioxide, or sulfites.
8. **Lupin**- ground or seeds, lupin flours or powders; lupin butters, oils, or sauces, lupin paste or nut meat, lupine or extract, lupin protein or pulp, lupin boiled or fibrous, lupin seasons or substitutes.
9. **Sesame**- ground or seeds, sesame oil or gingelly oil, benne seed, sesame leaf or sprouts; sesame flours, salt, or sauce.
10. **Mustard**- ground or seeds, mustard seasons or powder, mustard leaves or sprouts; mustard butters, oils, or sauces.
11. **Gluten**- flours or powders, cakes or sweet breads, Tortillas, bread or biscuits, seasons or packets, butters, sauces, or oils, protein packages, refined foods, processed foods. Gluten species include: wheat, durum wheat, semolina, spelt, kamut, einkorn, faro, barley, rye, oat, malt, couscous and mixes of these.
12. **Dairy**- milk or buttermilk, milk solids or derivatives, curds or cultured milk, condensed or evaporated, powders or dried milk, fat-free, %, or skim milk, creams even sweet ones, goat's or lamb milk, malted milk or whey, milk, proteins or casein, pasteurized milk, whipped cream, sour cream or pastes, butter, extract, or fat, butter flavored oils, butter solids or derivative; cheese cottage, or yogurt; cream cheese or cheese, imitation cheese, vegetarian cheeses, Custard or pudding, Galactose, or Lactalbumin.
13. **Celery**- ground or seeds, celery seasons or powder, celery leaves or sprouted; celery butters, oils, or sauces, celery salts, Celeriac root or stalk.
14. **Tree Nuts**- ground or seeds, nut flours or powders; nut butters, oils, or sauces; nut paste or nut meat, nut kernels or peas, nut protein or pulp, nuts boiled or cold pressed, nuts extruded or expelled, nut syrup or nut extract. Tree nut species include: almond, walnuts, brazil nuts, anacardium, shea nuts, pecans, hazelnuts, cashews, macadamia, pistachios, butternuts, and etc.

Detoxes and Remedies

Detoxes and Remedies

Hepatic Remedies

Liver Diseases

Complications with the liver can be serious. Viral infections along with alcoholism are the leading cause of dysfunction. Hepatic conditions can cause many nutritional complications, short term dysfunction, or severe malnutrition. This is why routine detoxification is important.

Symptoms of can be recognized within hours. A person can experience fatigue, severe weakness, or upper abdominal pain. These are clear signs of malfunction. Also, manifestations that occur can be misleading and people may mistake symptoms for other health related problems.

Liver disease are often overlooked because high levels of carbohydrates/excess sugars; high consumptions of saturated lipids, trans fats, or hydrogenated oils; alcohol; and excess proteins are often the cause of many nutritional complications. People have so many varying implications, it is often hard to pinpoint liver malfunction.

Other Hepatic Conditions
Portal hypertension and primary biliary cirrhosis are common. Limiting proinflammatory foods to a minimal amount and removing alcohol, providing nutritional support can quickly produce positive results. Weight loss, consumption of water and addition of omega 3 fatty acids can also support liver function.

Therapeutic Herbs

- Dandelion Root
- Vervain
- Baldo
- Butternut
- Barberry
- Wahoo
- Wild Yam
- Golden Seal
- Balmony
- Fringetree Bark
- Milk Thistle

Detoxes and Remedies

Daily Therapeutic Approach

Therapeutic Approach 1:
All Hepatic Conditions should remove alcohol, caffeine, and supplement:

- Vitamin C
- Vitamin E
- Zinc
- Selenium
- Milk Thistle

Therapeutic Approach 2:
Hepatic Conditions with acute Inflammation are recommend by evidence-based studies to use all of the nutrients from Therapeutic Approach 1 and in addition:

- Cilantro Parsley Tea, suggested for vitamin A supplement
- Licorice Root

Therapeutic Approach 3:
Non Fatty Alcoholic Liver Disease are recommend by evidence-based studies to use all of the nutrients from Therapeutic Approach 1 and in addition:

- Basil Tea, suggested as a magnesium supplement
- 2 hard boiled eggs, suggested for choline supplement

Other Considerations

When people begin eating healthy some will abruptly disinclude healthy fats. This increases their risk of gallbladder issues. Detoxing the liver properly and in combination with the galbladder can help preserve hepatic function.

Gallbladder Diseases

Gallstones are an American disease produced by long term gallbladder disease. Gallstones are usually caused by eating the Standard American Diet (SAD). Gallstones are caused by delayed gallbladder emptying, accelerated nucleation of cholesterol monohydrate in bile, supersaturation of bile with cholesterol. Other factors such as obesity, lipid lowering drugs, alcohol abuse, drug abuse, food sensitivities that increase symptoms, a decrease in water soluble vitamins, and lifestyle issues can also cause stress on this organ.

Foods that cause gallstones to worsen are egg, pork, milk, coffee, beans, sugar, and nuts. Botanicals such as taraxacum, peumus, silybum, Cynara, and curcuma which increase bile flow from liver; vitamins C and E are highly recommended along with 8 oz of pur water every hour, methionine also increases bile flow of liver, to dissolve gallstones simply adopt a vegetarian diet

Other Gallbladder Conditions
Sclerosing cholangitis, cholecystitis, gallstones as well as, gallbladder disease are considered dysfunctions of the gallbladder. They are caused by the excess consumption of refined carbohydrates, processed foods, hydrogenated fats and oils, fried foods, dairy products, and gluten products.

Therapeutic Nutrients
- Dandelion Root
- Barberry
- Baldo
- Fringetree Bark
- Goldenseal
- Balmony

Therapeutic Approach
Cholagogues are suggested for gallbladder diseases, they can be combined with butternut or wild yams, and supplement:
- Vitamin C
- Vitamin E
- Lethicin
- Milk Thistle
- Fish oil
- Reduce the amount of protein eaten

Meal Plans and Menus

What exactly is a Detoxification Diet?

A detoxification diet is a is a diet that can be personalized to improve the health an individual. There is no 1-size fits all approach to implementing a detox protocol. Each person is different with different circumstances, and although a foundation can be built, and a structure can be followed, each person must tweak their detox routine along the way.

How To Prepare

Cooking Conversions	
Cooking conversions help make it easier to learn portion sizes. They are also great for recipe preparation.	
Measurements	**Description**
1 Tablespoon (Tbsp)	15 Milliliters (ml) or 3 Teaspoons (tsp)
1 Ounce (oz)	T28.35 Grams (g), 29.57 Milliliters (ml), 2 Tablespoons (Tbsp), or 6 Teaspoons (tsp)
1 Cup (c)	8 Ounces (oz) or 16 Tablespoons (tbsp)
1 Pint (pt)	1 Pounds (lb), 2 Cups (c), or 16 Ounces (oz)
1 Quart (qt)	0.95 Liters (L), 2 Pints (pt), 2 Pounds (lb), 4 Cups (c), or 32 Ounces (oz)
1 Liter	1.05 Quarts (qt), 2.11 Pints (pt), or 4.16 Cups (c)
1 Gallon	3.8 Liters (L), 4 Quarts (qt), 8 Pints (pt), 8 Pounds (lb), 16 Cups (c), or 128 Ounces (oz)
Extras:	1 Teaspoon is 5 Milliliters (ml) 1 Pound is 454 Grams (g) 1 kilogram is 2.2 lbs 1 Liter is 1.05 Quarts (qt) 1 Peck is 2 Gallons (gal) 1 Bushel is 4 Pecks
Tools	
Hamilton Beach, 4-Quart Slow Cooker, silver; Model # 33443	
Know Your Foods	
Recipes are seasoned with vegetables and herbs that provide nutrients; robust, umami savory, and bitters flavors; and alkalizing hepatic, galactagogue, cholagogue, and bitters properties.	
Know The Rules	
1. Detoxify 2. Hydrate 3. Add Antioxidants	

Independent Meal Planning

Serving sizes are dependent on calorie needs.

Items	Pick at least 3	Pick at least 3	Pick at least 3	Pick 1-2 if desired
Meal	Breakfast	Lunch	Dinner	Snack
Fruit	½ cup berries of various colors	1/2 cup or 1 medium fruit		1/2 cup or 1 medium fruit
Protein	Lean animal or plant protein sources 2-3 servings	Lean animal protein 4-5 oz	Lean animal protein 4-5 oz	Bone broth, or plant protein shake
Healthy fats	1 oz nuts/seeds, or 2 tbsp oils or ½ half avocado		1 oz nuts/seeds, or 2 tbsp oils or ½ half avocado	1 oz nuts/seeds, 1 avocado
Non-dairy alternatives	Coconut, almond, soy, flaxseed, hemp, oat, or cashew	Coconut, almond, soy, flaxseed, hemp, oat, or cashew	Coconut, almond, soy, flaxseed, hemp, oat, or cashew	Coconut, almond, soy, flaxseed, hemp, oat, or cashew
Non-starchy vegetables	1-2 cups greens, varied, colorful	2 cups greens, varied, colorful	2 cups greens, varied, colorful	1 cup greens, varied, colorful
Starchy Carbs	1-2 servings whole grain high nutrient density	1-2 servings whole grain, high nutrient density		

Therapeutic Food Options

Type	Description
Meat	Grass-fed, and hormone free if possible Beef, buffalo, elk, lamb, venison, other wild game
Poultry/Eggs	Free range, caged free, or hormone free if possible
Protein Powder	Egg, Hemp, pea, rice, soy, whey (dependent on dairy sensitivity or not)
Plant based protein	Bean, mushroom, soy, veggie, tofu or tempeh
Fruits	Organic, non- GMO, colorful, and ripe if possible: Apple, blackberries, blueberries, cherries, grapefruit, mandarins, orange, pineapple, pomegranate seeds, raspberries, strawberries, tangerines
Vegetables	Organic, non- GMO, green, colorful, and ripe if possible ***Cruciferous family***: arugula, broccoflower, broccoli, broccoli sprouts, Brussel sprouts, cabbage, cauliflower, horseradish, kohlrabi, radishes ***Detoxifying Leafy Greens***: bok choy, chard/swiss chard, chervil, cilantro, endive, escarole, greens (beet, collard, dandelion, kale, mustard, turnip), microgreens, parsley, radicchio ***Thiols family***: chives, daikon radishes, garlic, leeks, onion, scallions, shallots ***Liver and Kidney support***: artichokes, asparagus, celeriac root, celery, all sprouts
Grains/Starches	Organic and non- GMO if possible Beets, black cooked soybeans, edamame, rolled or steel-cut oats, quinoa, buckwheat/Kasha, millet
Fats, Nuts, & Seeds, Oils	Non-hydrogenated, cold-pressed, organic, non-GMO if possible ***Fats:*** avocado, olives, coconut, palm fruit ***Nuts/Seeds:*** almonds, brazil nuts, cashews, chia seeds, coconut unsweetened dried flakes, ground flaxseed, hemp seeds, nut and seed butters, mixed nuts, pecans, pine nuts, pistachios, pumpkin seeds, sunflower seed kernels, sesame seeds, soy nuts, walnuts ***Cooking Oils:*** coconut, olive (extra virgin), sesame ***Oils for Salad:*** flaxseed, olive (extra virgin), rice bran, sesame

7-Day Detoxification Menu

Serving sizes are dependent on calorie needs.

Day	Breakfast	Lunch	Dinner	Snack
1	Steel cut oats with flaxseed, walnuts, blueberries, with coconut milk. Can add in a plant protein or eggs for additional protein.	Grilled chicken with stir fry vegetables over quinoa	Grass-fed sirloin with mixed california steamed vegetables and sweet potato	2 small tangerines
2	Overnight oats with coconut kefir, chia seeds, raspberries, almond slivers, 1 tsp raw honey and 1/2 tsp cinnamon	4 vegetable edamame soup (made with any 4 vegetables of different colors) with beef bone broth and soy beans (edamame)	Turkey tenderloin roasted in olive oil, with rosemary, basil, thyme, and mustard seeds, with black rice, and brussel sprouts	Small handful of pistachios, almonds, and brazil nuts
3	Chicken egg scramble with onion, garlic, collard and dandelion greens with everything bagel seasoning, himalayan salt, pepper, and chopped turmeric root	Tofu with broccoli and sauteed greens using olive oil, garlic, scallions, bok choy, mushrooms, and tumeric root over black rice	Bison burger (made at home with fine chopped onions, garlic, and ginger with favorite spices) over sauteed mixed leafy greens and asparagus	1 cup pineapple in coconut yogurt with pomegranate seeds
4	Bone broth or plant protein smoothie with mixed berries, 1/2 avocado, 1/2 apple	Cabbage soup cooked with onion, celery, carrots, small potatoes, diced tomatoes, garlic, olive oil, organic chicken broth, spices to taste	Salmon over roasted artichoke made with olive oil, red onion, garlic cloves, lemon juice, black pepper, salt, and capers. Roast in a drizzle of fresh lemon juice, honey, fresh dill plus the garlic cloves.	1 cup cherries with 1 oz mixed nuts
5	Baked Egg muffins with garlic, onion, chopped bell peppers, spinach, 1 cup melon	Salmon over sauteed mixed dark greens over brown rice with sesame oil, rice vinegar, and olive oil	Ground chicken taco meat with avocado, chopped greens, onions, salsa, and olive oil on brown rice cakes	1 small apple
6	Sauteed spinach with eggs, tofu, onion, sesame seeds, olive oil scramble over quinoa	Black soy bean with quinoa soup and large mixed greens with arugula salad, pumpkin seeds, sesame seeds, walnuts, almonds, and watercress	Grilled chicken with roasted beets over red quinoa	Mixed fresh berries in soy yogurt, chia seeds, flaxseed, and raisins
7	Smoothie with coconut or almond milk, ginger, lemon, frozen mixed berries, mango, walnuts, 1 cup kale, cinnamon, nutmeg, and vanilla extract	Baked wild caught halibut with small red potatoes plus green beans sauteed with olive oil, garlic, salt, pepper, slivered almonds	Tofu roasted with broccoli, cauliflower, kohlrabi, bok choy, radicchio, endive, cilantro, arugula using olive oil and favorite spices	1/2 grapefruit

Meal Plans and Menus 57

7-Day Low-Sulfur Menu

Serving sizes are dependent on calorie needs.

7- Day Meal Planning Low Sulfur Diet

Day	Breakfast	Lunch	Dinner	Snack
1	Sweet potatoes cooked in olive oil, sea salt, and fresh herbs.	Red rice and beans, with sauteed spinach in olive oil with added sea salt.	Grilled stir fry veggies, such as zucchini, yellow squash, bell peppers and over brown rice with teriyaki sauce	Melon slices with cinnamon and pecans.
2	Oats with rice kefir, chia seeds, blueberries cashew slivers, and 1 tsp raw honey, ¼ tsp cinnamon, and ¼ tsp nutmeg.	Pumpkin soup with quinoa on the side and toasted sunflower seeds.	Large garden salad- romaine lettuce, tomato, cucumber, kalamata olives, banana peppers non-mustard vinaigrette.	Red apple with macadamia nut butter.
3	Juice/ Smoothie Equal parts of cucumber, gold beet, and celery. And 1 green apple.	Vegan stuffed tomatoes with couscous, peas, sweet potatoes, turnip cubes olive oils, and sea salt,	Ginger flavored baked asparagus with very small portion of halibut fish, and quinoa.	1 cup pineapple with black berries.
4	Juice/ Smoothie ¼ avocado, ½ banana, 6 macadamia nuts, ¼ tsp, cinnamon honey to taste, and pea protein powder.	Tomato soup cooked with gluten-free organic bread slices and cashew cheese to make grilled cheese sandwiches.	Very small portion of red snapper over roasted artichoke made with olive oil, lemon juice, black pepper, salt, and capers.	1 cup cherries with 1 oz macadamia nuts.
5	Red potatoes and mixed bell peppers cooked in olive oil, sea salt, fresh garlic, and fresh herbs.	Very small portion of salmon with sauteed yellow squash over brown rice.	Vegan taco salad with romaine lettuce, corn, black beans, avocado, over grilled bell peppers and brown rice.	Green apple with cashew nut butter.
6	Steel cut oats with flaxseed, walnuts, blueberries, with flax milk.	Grilled portobello mushroom, brushed with olive oil, sea salt, pepper, basil over roasted potatoes.	Zoodles and organic made spaghetti sauce, with sauteed tomato halves.	2 small tangerines
7	Juice/ Smoothie Equal parts of 6 strawberries, ¼ cup of cranberries, ¼ red beet, and ½ cup raspberries.	Baked red potatoes in olive oil with rosemary, sea salt; served with green beans and slivered hazelnuts.	Cashew cheese stuffed mushrooms, toasted pumpkin seeds, with peas and carrots.	½ grapefruit

Meal Plans and Menus

7-Day Triple C Menu

Clearing Cellular Congestion

Serving sizes are dependent on calorie needs.

Day	Breakfast	Lunch	Dinner
1	Chamomile Tea Cabbage Soup Strawberries Vitamin E	Hydrogen-rich Water Tomato Soup Goat cheese Whole grain crackers	Hydrogen-rich Water Shrimp/pineapple kabobs Zucchini Seaweed Salad
2	Turmeric Tea Dandelion Leaf Soup Dried Cranberries Ascorbic Acid	Ginger Lemonade Cabbage Soup Avocado Fermented Artichokes	Hydrogen-rich Water Baked Chicken Butternut Squash
3	Green Tea Pumpkin Soup Blackberries Glutathione	Hydrogen-rich Water Dandelion Leaf Soup Avocado Fermented Beets	Hydrogen-rich Water Lemon Caper Trout Sauteed Spinach Sunflower Seeds
4	Hydrogen-rich Water Tomato Soup Grapefruit B-complex	Cherry Limeade Pumpkin Soup 6 Olives Fermented Banana Peppers	Hydrogen-rich Water Baked Pork Ribs Green beans Sauteed Almondine
5	Hibiscus/Passion Tea Cabbage Soup Raspberries Vitamin E	Almond Lemonade Tomato Soup Goat cheese Whole grain crackers	Hydrogen-rich Water Peanut/pumpkin chicken Cauliflower rice
6	Black Tea Dandelion Leaf Soup Mango Ascorbic Acid	Hydrogen-rich Water Cabbage Soup Avocado Fermented Artichokes	Hydrogen-rich Water Ground beef Mushroom sauce Rice
7	Hydrogen-rich Water Pumpkin Soup Blueberries Glutathione	Basil Ginger Limeade Dandelion Leaf Soup Avocado Fermented Beets	Hydrogen-rich Water Turkey wing Quinoa Bean/corn mix

Recipes

Recipes

Lunch Juice Detox: Taste the Rainbow
- Whole raw cranberries or raspberries, 1/2 cup
- Golden beetroot, 1/2 root (F, P)
- Golden beet greens, 1/4 cup of bundle from 1 root
- Spinach, 1/4 cup
- Blueberries or black berries, 1/2 cup

Instructions: Blend everything in the bullet.

Detox Information: Beetroot and leaves, spinach, cranberries, raspberries, blackberries, and blueberries help increase fiber, phytonutrients, and omega 3 fatty acids needed for detox.

Detox Turmeric Tea

By: Jasmine Hollywood

Find the blend at https://www.jasmineblake.com/coastal-vibes-holistic-blends
Or- use your own!

Instructions:
Add 50mg of turmeric to 8 oz of steaming water. Recommended amount 1x/q.d.

Title	Description
Name	Also known as Curcuma longa, and from the ginger family, Zingiberaceae can be used as anti-inflammatory (Alok et al., 2015). It is also known to be anti-carcinogenic, antiperoxidant, hepatoprotective, a metal chelator, a Cox-2 inhibitor, anti-nitrososaminic, and antiangiogenic, amongst many other anti properties (Alok et al., 2015).
Function	Tumeric has a strong affinity for scavenging superoxide radicals, hydrogen peroxide and nitric oxide (NO) from activated macrophages, reducing iron complex and inhibiting lipid peroxidation (Alok et al., 2015). May be used to negatively and positively influence CYP1A2, CYP2B1, and CYP3A4 enzyme activity; enhance UGT activity, restore depleted GSH; and stimulate Nrf2 activity (Hodges, & Minich, 2015).
Recipe	The typical dose is a diet of 1% turmeric for influencing the activity of CYP1A2 and CYP2B1 enzymes and enhancing UGT activity; 50 and 100 mg/kg curcumin for influencing CYP3A4 activity, and 50 -200 mg/kg/d curcumin stimulate Nrf2 activity (Hodges, & Minich, 2015). One cup of tea with a 50mg solution per day is more than adequate.
Emotional Release	Journaling while drinking your tea in a quiet area!

Recipes

Limeades

Immune Boosters

Title	Ingredients
Basil Ginger Limeade	<ul><li>2 quarts of carbonated water</li><li>¼ cup of fresh Basil</li><li>2 inches Ginger root, chopped</li><li>½ cup Raw Organic Honey</li><li>¾ cup of fresh squeezed lime juice</li><li>1 Lime, sliced</li></ul> **Instructions:** Pour the lime juice and the raw organic honey in a dish and whisk together. Then pour into container. Add water and mix.Do not shake or it will fizz! Then add ginger, basil, and lime slices. Let sit for 1 day. Batch is ready. Add honey to preferred taste. Refrigerate up to 1 week and no more.
Cherry Limeade	<ul><li>2 quarts of carbonated water</li><li>¼ cup of fresh cherries smashed</li><li>½ cup Raw Organic Honey</li><li>¾ cup of fresh squeezed lime juice</li><li>1 Lime, sliced</li></ul> **Instructions:** Pour the lime juice and the raw organic honey in a dish and whisk together. Then pour into container. Add water and mix. Do not shake or it will fizz! Then add cherries and the juices from being smashed. Let sit for 1 day. Batch is ready. Add honey to preferred taste. Refrigerate up to 1 week and no more.

Recipes

Lemonades

Immune Boosters

Title	Ingredients
Ginger Lemonade	<ul><li>2 quarts of water</li><li>⅓ cup of fresh squeezed lemon juice</li><li>1 Lemon, sliced</li><li>2 inches Ginger root, sliced</li><li>½ cup Raw Organic Honey</li></ul>**Instructions:** Pour the lemon juice and the raw organic honey in a dish and whisk together. Then pour into container. Add water and mix, or shake. Then add ginger and lemon slices. Let sit for 1 day. Batch is ready. Add honey to preferred taste. Refrigerate up to 1 week and no more.
Almond Lemonade	<ul><li>2 quarts of water</li><li>⅓ cup of fresh squeezed lemon juice</li><li>1 Lemon, sliced</li><li>1-2 ounces of almond extract</li><li>½ cup Raw Organic Honey</li></ul>**Instructions:** Pour the lemon juice and the raw organic honey in a dish and whisk together. Then pour into container. Add water and mix, or shake. Then add almond extract and lemon slices. Let sit for 1 day. Batch is ready. Add honey to preferred taste. Refrigerate up to 1 week and no more.

Dandelion and Cabbage Soups

Dandelion Soup

Ingredients

- ⅓ cup cashews
- 1 bunch dandelion greens (6 cups chopped)
- 4 large garlic cloves, chopped
- 1 yellow onion, chopped
- 2 cups cauliflower, blended
- 2 stalks celery chopped
- 4 cup vegetable stock
- 1 tbsp celtic sea salt
- ½ tsp black pepper
- 1 tbsp EVOO

Instructions:
Put all ingredients into crock pot. Seal container. Cook for 8 to 12 hours, stirring occasionally.

Considerations

Eat with vitamin C and avocado.

Probiotic and Gut Healer

Ingredients

- 1 head Green Cabbage
- 4 garlic cloves
- 1 small purple onion, chopped
- 1 tsp Sea Salt
- 1 tsp fresh Thyme
- 1 tsp fresh Rosemary
- 1 pkt Coastal Vibes Turmeric
- Chicken

Instructions:
Put all ingredients into a crock pot and make sure they fit well. You may even have extra room. Add water up until it reaches the top. Seal container. Cook for up to 24 hours, stirring occasionally.
Add chicken if you are a meat eater.

Considerations

Eat with vitamin E and avocado.

Recipes

Pumpkin and Tomato Soups

Pumpkin Soup

Ingredients

- Pumpkin puree
- Pumpkin seeds
- Green onions
- Unsweetened almond milk
- 7 garlic cloves
- 1 yellow onion

Instructions:
Put all ingredients into crock pot and make sure they fit well. You may even have extra room. Seal container. Cook up to 8 hours, stirring occasionally. Top with pumpkin seeds.

Considerations

Eat with glutathione, fermented banana peppers, and olives.

Tomato Soup

Ingredients

- 1 cup cherry tomatoes
- 2 large roma tomatoes, quarterd
- 1 can tomato paste
- 1 oz white onion, chopped
- 5 garlic cloves, chopped
- 1 stick celery, minced
- Vegetable stock
- 2 tsp Sea Salt
- 1 tsp dried parsley
- ½ tsp ground blakc pepper
- 1 tbsp EVOO

Instructions:
Put all ingredients into crock pot and make sure they fit well. You may even have extra room. Add water up until it reaches the consistency you desire. Seal container. Cook up to 8 hours, stirring occasionally.

Considerations

Eat with b-complex, goat cheese and whole grain crackers.

Recipes

Grapefruit Fennel Salad

Immune Booster

Ingredients

- 1 cup chopped Kale rubbed in: 1 tbsp of sunflower oil
- ¼ cup of almonds
- ⅛ cup of sunflower seeds
- ½ small grapefruit supreme'd
- ½ cup fresh fennel tips roughly chopped
- ¼ cup yellow squash thinly sliced

Instructions:
SAUCE
Squeeze other half of grapefruit into bowl & add ¼ tsp sea salt, ½ garlic clove, 1 chopped chive, 1 small dash of white wine vinegar, chopped cauliflower, 2 almonds sliced, 3 large strawberries, 3 peppercorns. Blend.
PLATE
Add all the prepared ingredients together. Pour sauce over the ingredients. Ready to serve.

Considerations

Eat with b-complex, goat cheese and whole grain crackers.

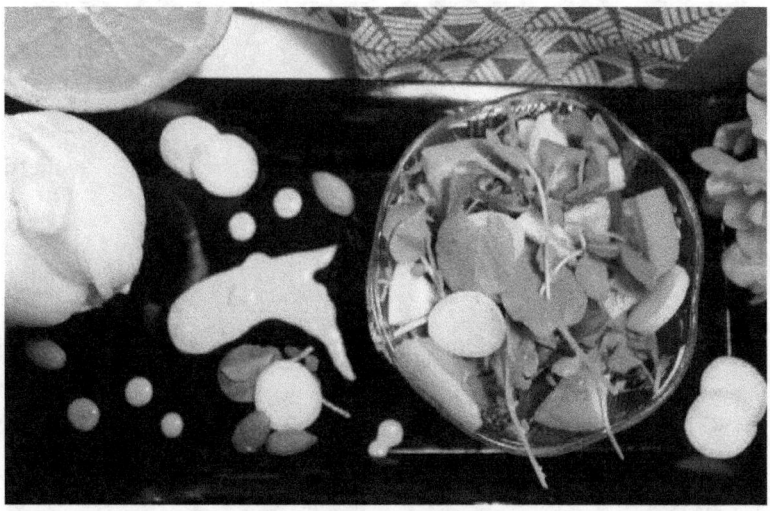

Baked Artichokes

Detox Booster

Ingredients

- 1 bag of jerusalem artichokes
- ½ cup onion, sliced
- 1 cup frozen peas
- ¼ cup avocado oil
- 1 tbsp rosemary
- 1 tbsp thyme
- 1 tbsp sea salt
- 6 whole garlic cloves
- 1 tbsp sage
- 2 cups of water

Instructions:
In a glass baking pan place the artichokes, peas, onions and garlic inside. Turn oven on 350 degrees F. Sprinkle herbs and sea salt on top. Drizzle oil over the food. Pour water inside, cover with aluminum foil and place inside oven.

After 2 hours, take out food. Stir it around. Puree in blender a little bit at a time. After all is pureed, it is ready to serve. Can sprinkle some herbs on top for look.

Good for 2 days in refrigerator.

Considerations

Eat with ascorbic acid, mixed fruit, or hydrogen rich water.

Porterhouse Chops

Gut and Organ Healer

Ingredients

- 1 porterhouse pork chop
- ¼ cup sliced mushrooms
- ¼ cup sliced onion
- ¼ cup chopped cilantro
- 2 tbsp safflower oil
- pinch of dill, mixed with peppercorns
- tbsp of rosemary
- 1 tbsp red wine vinegar
- 1 sliced garlic clove
- ¼ tsp cumin

Instructions:
Saute pork chop on medium heat in safflower oil. Add mushrooms and onion and cook until translucent. Add other ingredients and saute until done. Ready to serve.

Considerations

Eat with b-complex, over rice.

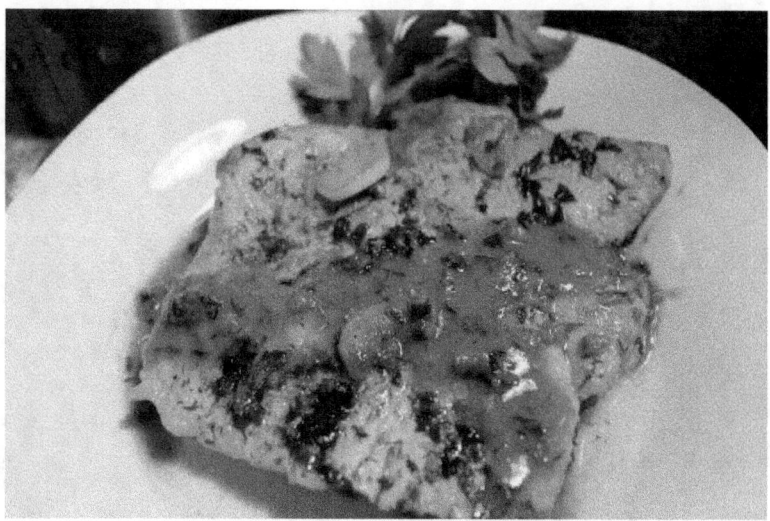

Chipotle Salsa

Immune Booster

Ingredients

- 2 cups mixed chopped bell peppers, seeded and gutted
- 1 chipotle chopped, seeded and gutted
- 3 garlic cloves, minced
- ¼ cup dried red peppers
- 1 jalapenos, seeded and gutted
- ½ cup purple onion, chopped
- ½ cup cilantro, finely chopped
- ¼ cup lime juice
- 1 tsp Coastal Vibes Seasoning
- ½ tbsp salt

Instructions:
Pulse all the ingredients in blender or bullet but do not puree. Leave some whole pieces.

Add all the ingredients together in a sealed tight 2 part lid - 2 qrt. container. Let ferment in refrigerator for 3 days. After 3 days is up, it is ready to serve.

As long as it's in container sealed, it can be good up to 2 weeks.

Considerations

Eat with b-complex, goat cheese and whole grain crackers.

Recipes

Asparagus Almondine

Vitamin E Booster

Ingredients

- bundle of asparagus
- ½ cup of almonds, sliced
- 2 tbsp sunflower seed oil
- 1 tsp sea salt
- 2 garlic cloves sliced
- ¼ cup white onions

Instructions:
Saute asparagus with sunflower seed oil and ½ tsp of sea salt. Empty out of pan. Use same pan without washing. Add the onions and garlic, cook until onions are translucent. Then add almonds, and rest of salt. Saute until almonds are soft and browned. Pour over asparagus. Ready to serve.

Considerations

Eat with b-complex, goat cheese and whole grain crackers.

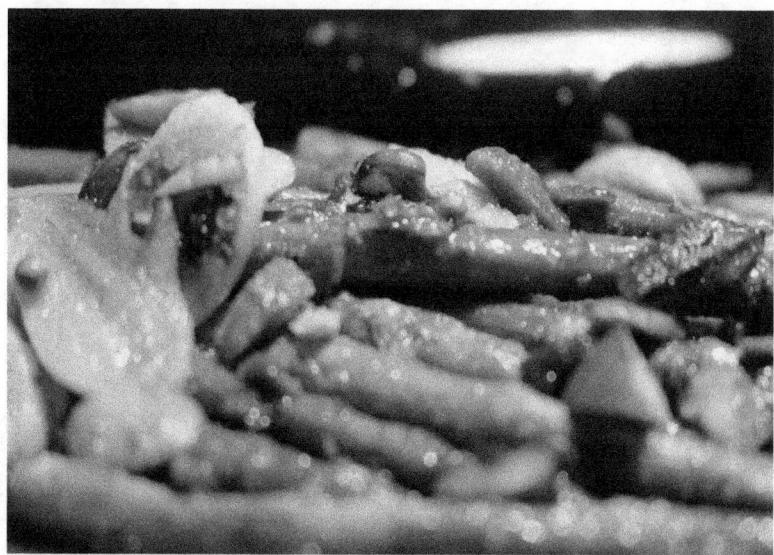

Extras

Extras

Nutrition Booster Tips

Cooking Meats and Starches

Steak
Sear steak with 1 sliced garlic clove, 2 tbsp sliced chives, dash of coriander, ¼ tsp sunflower seed oil with a pinch of sea salt and pepper.

Potatoes
On the side bake or boil 4 small red potatoes sliced and tossed in dill, sunflower seed oil, and pinch of sea salt. Ready to serve.

Lamb
Sear lamb quickly on medium heated pan then set to bake in a baking pan. Then, cook rice in a 2 qrt pot, and when done with rice, add ¼ cup lime juice, fresh chopped cilantro or parsley, and 1 tbsp sea salt.

Pork
Bake pork in a baking pan rubbed with the following combination: a pinch of rosemary, dash of paprika, 1 garlic clove minced. On the side mix ¼ cup thinly slice red cabbage, dash or 2 of white wine vinegar, and add red bell peppers and purple onions. Bake with pork or eat cabbage mix fresh.

Rice
Cook rice in a 1 qt pot and when done add ½ tbsp sea salt, ⅛ cup of lemon juice, 1 tbsp of chopped chives. In a pot cook 1 cup of any kind of beans or legumes and add 1 tbsp safflower oil, 1 tbsp purple onions, garlic to taste, sea salt to taste and pepper. Ready to serve.

Ground Beef
Bake ground beef mixed with ½ cup peas, brussels sprouts, 2, tbsp yeast, 2 tbsp purple onion, ½ stalk of leeks sliced, 2 tbsp safflower oil, a dash fennel, a dash sage, 1 tsp ground garlic, 5 crushed kalamata olives, 7 peppercorns, ¼ tsp salt, 1 tsp white wine vinegar, and 1 tbsp herbs of Provence.7

Extras

Antioxidant Smoothies

Oxidation Thieves

Bloody Mary
- ¼ cup kale, 1 large tomato, ⅛ cup green pepper, ¼ cup red cabbage, 1 small garlic clove, 7 peppercorns, ⅛ tsp salt, 3 large green olives, ¼ lime squeezed, ⅛ tsp onion powder.

The Diamond In the Rough
- ⅓ red banana, 4 peanuts, ⅓ plantain, 2 almonds, 1 tbsp of sunflower seeds, and ½ bar 70% cocoa.

Water Woman
- (hydrogen rich) ¼ cup watermelon, ¼ cup cantaloupe, ¼ cup pineapple, ½ peach, and 1 apricot.

Berry Mary Quite Contrary
- (antioxidant rich) ¼ cup blueberries, ¼ cup raspberries, ¼ cup strawberries, and ¼ cup blackberries.

The Riddler
- 1 kiwi, ½ cup pineapple, ½ cup honeydew melon, ¼ cup yellow bell peppers, and ½ green apple.

Iron Man
- ¼ cup mustard greens, 1 green apple, 2 celery stalks, ¼ cup kale, dash of sage, and ¼ cup spinach.

Caribbean Queen
- ¼ cup papaya, ¼ cup soursop, ¼ cup mango, and ¼ cup passion fruit.

Alice in Switzerland
- ¼ cup cherries, 1 plum, ¼ cup blackberries, 1 apricot, and ¼ cup red apple

Cruciferous of All
- ¼ cup broccoli, ¼ cup cauliflower, ¼ cup brussel sprouts, ¼ cup asparagus tips, ¼ cucumber, and 2 kiwis.

References

References

Al-Mamary, M. A. , & Moussa, Z. (2021). Antioxidant Activity: The Presence and Impact of Hydroxyl Groups in Small Molecules of Natural and Synthetic Origin. In (Ed.), Antioxidants - Benefits, Sources, Mechanisms of Action.

Ask the Oracle [vitamin and nutrient summary for recipes]. (2019). *Cronometer Pro*.

Blake, J. (2018). Cranberry Tomatillo Salsa [Image]. Retrieved from Discover Your Greatest Self Archives.

Blake, J. (2018). Grapefruit Fennel Salad [Image]. Retrieved from Discover Your Greatest Self Archives.

Blake, J. (2018). Asparagus Almondine [Image]. Retrieved from Discover Your Greatest Self Archives.

Blake, J. (2018).Porterhouse Pork Chop [Image]. Retrieved from Discover Your Greatest Self Archives.

Blake, J. (2018). All Recipes and Food Combinations [Recipes]. Retrieved from Discover Your Greatest Self Archives.

Boyer J. L. (2013). Bile formation and secretion. *Comprehensive Physiology*, *3*(3), 1035–1078. doi:10.1002/cphy.c120027

Digestive Diseases. (n.d.). *National Institute of Diabetes and Digestive and Kidney diseases*.

Freedman, B. J. (1980). Sulphur dioxide in foods and beverages: its use as a preservative and its effect on asthma. British Journal of Diseases of the Chest. 74(2), 128-34.

Gaby, A. R. (2017). *Nutritional medicine (2nd ed.)*. Concord, NH: Fritz Perlberg Publishing.

Hodges, R. E. & Minich, D. M. (2015). Modulation of metabolic detoxification pathways using foods and food-derived components: A scientific review with clinical application. *Journal of Nutrition and Metabolism*.

Lieberman, M., & Peet, A. (2018). *Mark's basic medical biochemistry: A clinical approach (5th ed.)*. Philadelphia, PA: Wolters Kluwer.

Lobo, V., Patil, A., Phatak, A., & Chandra, N. (2010). Free radicals, antioxidants and functional foods: Impact on human health. *Pharmacognosy reviews*, *4*(8), 118–126.

Mahan, L. K. & Raymond, J. L. (2014). *Krause's food and the nutrition care process (14th ed.)*. St. Louis, MO: Elsevier.

Masri, O. A., Chalhoub, J. M., & Sharara, A. I. (2015). Role of vitamins in gastrointestinal diseases. *World journal of gastroenterology*, *21*(17), 5191–5209. doi:10.3748/wjg.v21.i17.5191

Mulrow C, Lawrence V, Jacobs B, et al. (2000). *Milk thistle: Effects on liver disease and cirrhosis and clinical adverse effects: Summary...* In: AHRQ Evidence Report Summaries, 1998-2005, 21. Rockville (MD): Agency for Healthcare Research and Quality (US).

NMDF211: Nutritional Biochemistry, Liver detoxification pathways: Session 6 [PDF]. (n.d.). Endeavour College of Natural Health.

References

Onanuga, K., Begley, U., & Begley, T. J. (2016). Understanding the role of selenium in Reactive oxygen species management in colorectal cancers. *Free Radical Biology and Medicine, 100,* S127-S128.

Phang-Lyn S, Llerena VA. Biochemistry, Biotransformation. [Updated 2021 Aug 30]. In: StatPearls [Internet]. Treasure Island (FL): StatPearls Publishing; 2022 Jan.

Phaniendra, A., Jestadi, D. B., & Periyasamy, L. (2015). Free radicals: properties, sources, targets, and their implication in various diseases. *Indian journal of clinical biochemistry : IJCB, 30*(1), 11–26.

Recipe Photos. (2019). *Dreams Time.*

Rice, A. (2018). Almond, Rosemary, & Basil Pesto [Image]. Retrieved from Discover Your Greatest Self Archives.

Rice, A. (2018). Spicy Pepper Salsa [Image]. Retrieved from Discover Your Greatest Self Archives.

Ross, A. C., Caballero, B., Cousins, R. J., Tucker, K. L., & Ziegler. (2014). *Modern Nutrition in Health and Disease, 11th Ed.* Philadelphia, PA: Wolters Kluwer.

Swallah, M. S., Sun, H., Affoh, R., Fu, H., & Yu, H. (2020). Antioxidant Potential Overviews of Secondary Metabolites (Polyphenols) in Fruits. *International journal of food science, 2020,* 9081686.

Traber, M. G., & Stevens, J. F. (2011). Vitamins C and E: beneficial effects from a mechanistic perspective. *Free radical biology & medicine, 51*(5), 1000–1013. doi:10.1016/j.freeradbiomed.2011.05.017

Walcher, T., Haenle, M. M., Kron, M., Hay, B., Mason, R. A., Walcher, D., ... EMIL study group (2009). Vitamin C supplement use may protect against gallstones: an observational study on a randomly selected population. *BMC gastroenterology, 9,* 74. doi:10.1186/1471-230X-9-74

Yasutake, K., Kohjima, M., Nakashima, M., Kotoh, K., Nakamuta, M., & Enjoji, M. (2012). Nutrition therapy for liver diseases based on the status of nutritional intake. *Gastroenterology Research and Practice, 2012,* 859697. doi:10.1155/2012/859697

Your digestive system and how it works. (2017). *National Institute of Diabetes and Digestive and Kidney diseases.*

Zhang, Y., Berman, G. P., & Kais, S. (2015). The radical pair mechanism and the avian chemical compass: Quantum coherence and entanglement. *The International Journal of Quantum Chemistry, 115*(19): 1327-1341.

www.ingramcontent.com/pod-product-compliance
Lightning Source LLC
Chambersburg PA
CBHW050141240426
43673CB00043B/1752